Keto Meal Prep for Beginners

Your Essential Ketogenic Diet Easy Meal Plan to Save Time & Money for Long-Term Weight Loss, Eating Better and Healthy Living (PLUS: Easy Meal Prep Ideas on a Budget)

Amy Maria Adams

© **Copyright 2019 by Amy Maria Adams - All rights reserved.**

The contents of this book may not be reproduced, duplicated or transmitted without direct written permission from the author.

Under no circumstances will any legal responsibility or blame be held against the publisher for any reparation, damages, or monetary loss due to the information herein, either directly or indirectly.

Legal Notice:

This book is copyright protected. This is only for personal use. You cannot amend, distribute, sell, use, quote or paraphrase any part or the content within this book without the consent of the author.

Disclaimer Notice:

Please note the information contained within this document is for educational and entertainment purposes only. Every attempt has been made to provide accurate, up to date and reliable complete information. No warranties of any kind are expressed or implied. Readers acknowledge that the author is not engaging in the rendering of legal, financial, medical or professional advice. The content of this book has been derived from various sources. Please consult a licensed professional before attempting any techniques outlined in this book.

By reading this document, the reader agrees that under no circumstances are is the author responsible for any losses, direct or indirect, which are incurred as a result of the use of information contained within this document, including, but not limited to, —errors, omissions, or inaccuracies.

Table of Contents

Introduction

Chapter 1: Getting Started with Keto Meal Prep Plan

Chapter 2: How to Begin Meal Prepping

Chapter 3: Easy Steps to Meal Prepping

Chapter 4: Simple Go-To Recipes to Start

Chapter 5: The Main Recipes

Chapter 6: Keto Meal Prep on a Budget

Chapter 7: Keto Meal Prep for Weight Loss

Chapter 8: Keto Meal Prep—Mistakes to Avoid

Bonus Chapter: Money-Savings Tips When Shopping

Conclusion

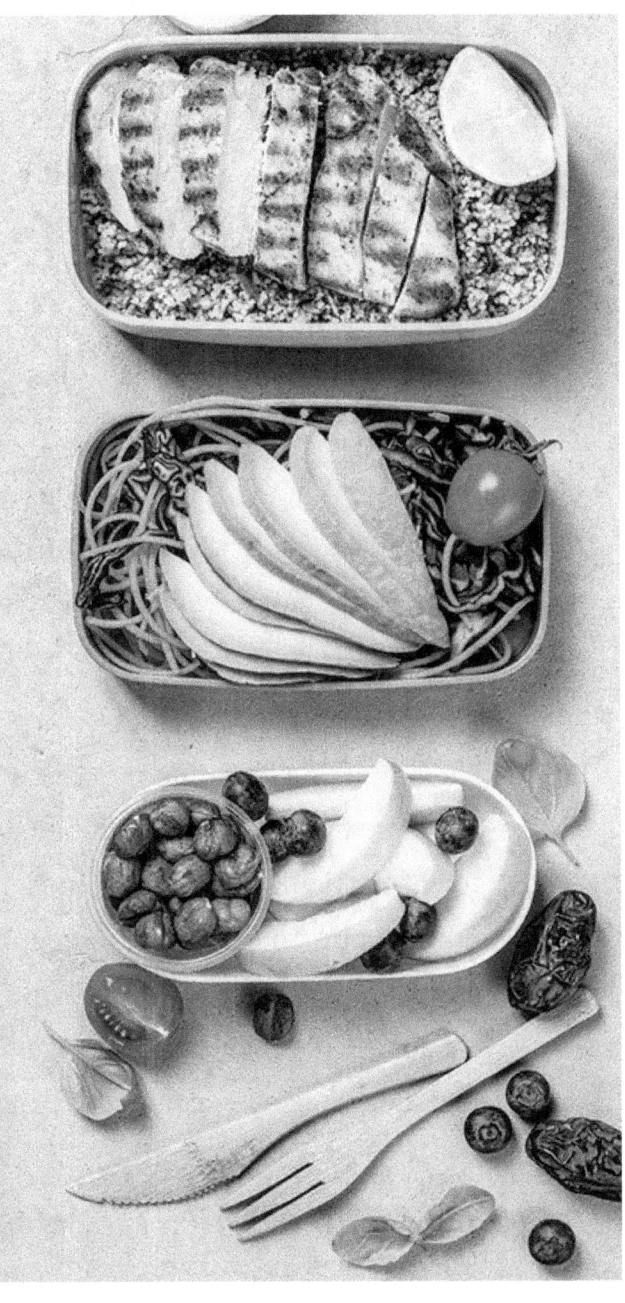

Introduction:

It is unfortunate to say, but sometimes we are so busy to think of what we want or should eat, let alone what we should cook. It is not very easy to eat healthy foods if you lead a busy life unless you have everything planned. *Deciding what to eat every day can, sadly, be a source of stress.* What you will cook for dinner or what you will eat for breakfast or lunch can get tiring, especially if you are on a healthy lifestyle.

Now, imagine for someone who is on a diet such as the keto diet, which demands that you have to eat particular foods for the right nutrition to power your body with sufficient energy! While many of us aspire to live healthy lifestyles and set goals to eat healthy, it is never easy following through, and consistency is a big problem. In fact, it is something as simple as having the right meals to eat, which makes many of us fall off the wagon. This is why meal prepping is a great concept for those on the ketogenic diet.

When you're busy navigating through your daily life, the thought of cooking all of your own meals at home can sometimes feel impossible. Not to mention warding off temptations at restaurants. And let's face it—time is the number-one "make or break" factor when it comes to deciding on a meal.

Those who are on a ketogenic diet know all too well that *it can be a tricky affair getting the food you like at an affordable price and which will not take a long time to prepare after a long day or even on those days when you just feel off.* Keto meal prepping ensures that you have the food as per your diet all the time—the question of what you should eat will never arise.

For somebody who may be wondering what a ketogenic diet is or someone who is looking for a great dieting option, *the keto diet focuses on foods that will get your body into a metabolic state of called ketosis, where the body burns fat for energy instead of carbs. In other words, you will be on a high-fat, low-carb diet to achieve weight loss or other dieting goals.*

The idea is based on the fact that most weight gain and fat accumulation in the body is as a result of high carbs intake. Carbohydrates are converted into glycogen and fat by the body. The glycogen is stored in the muscles, and the leftover converted carbs are stored as fat.

When the body is starved of new carbs, it burns up the glycogen stored in the muscles. Once exhausted, the body resorts to the fat reservoir for energy. It is for this reason that the ketogenic diet is so popular and is the most recommended diet for weight loss. It is essentially weight loss without opting out of some foods. You can eat virtually anything you want as long as it fits into the diet.

Ketosis has proven to have a variety of health benefits, which include weight loss, blood sugar regulation, disease management (diabetes, high blood pressure, cholesterol issues, etc.), and enhanced mental performance. Ketosis starves your body of carbohydrates, which the liver converts to glucose—reduced glucose means the body burns fat for energy.

Back to the topic at hand. *Meal prepping simply means preparing whole meals ahead of schedule so that they are available for you to eat when the time comes.* This concept is ideal for the busy lifestyle and has gained popularity with people for the amazing time-saving benefits and other benefits, which we will discuss later in this book.

Apart from having ready meals, this concept ensures that you eat reduces portion to help you reach your dieting goals. No more fast food because prepping guarantees that you eat more nutritious meals and no more late-night meals because you always have a ready dish.

The good thing about meal prepping is that you customize it to fit your availability and needs.

There is no standard method of doing it. Choose the day to prep your meals and switch it if you have to.

What about if you are reading this and you are not on a keto diet? Well, meal prepping is still something you should consider for the many benefits on offer. Everyone wants an easier life; therefore, meal planning can be adopted by all of us. Meal prep is not only for those on a keto diet; it can be adapted to fit any diet and lifestyle to guarantee that you will have a meal ready for you ahead of time.

By the end of this book, you will be well informed about meal prepping in general but, more specifically, keto meal prep. This book will cover the following:

- How to get started on keto prep meal plan
- Information on how to begin prepping
- Easy steps to meal prepping

- Simple breakfast, lunch, dinner, desserts, and snack keto recipes for beginners or anyone who wants a quick-fix meal
- Main keto recipes
- Keto meal prepping on a budget
- Meal prepping for weight loss
- Money-saving tips
- Measurement conversions

Meal prepping will simplify your life, save you a lot of time and money, and ensure that you live the healthy lifestyle you want by keeping you on track as far as eating healthy meals is concerned.

The answer to eating what you want affordably and without putting so much time and energy into cooking is meal prepping, and we shall give you great insights and share with you some great recipes to start you off.

Enjoy this introduction to meal prepping, the great recipes, and many other tips.

Chapter 1
Getting Started with Keto Meal Prep Plan

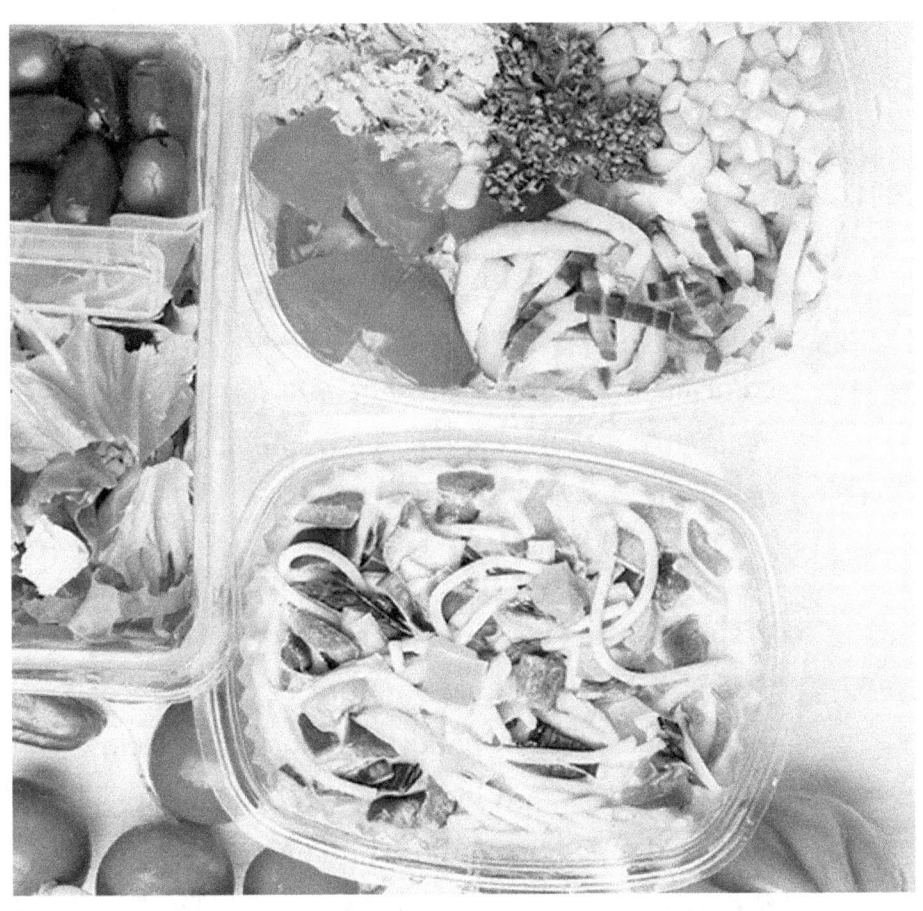

Chapter 1: Getting Started with Keto Meal Prep Plan

1.1 Definition of Keto Meal Prep Plan

We have touched on the meaning of a meal prep plan in the introduction and stated that it means to prepare meals in advance. *For the ketogenic diet, meal planning can be defined more specifically to mean preparing full meals in advance using keto approved ingredients, calories, and recipes so that you have meals ready to eat that meet the requirements of keto,* usually for a week.

The common and most convenient keto meal prep plan runs for a week. In other words, you will prepare meals for a whole week in advance on a designated day. Think about it, in one week, you will need twenty-one meals if you take three meals a day as you should. Thinking of the over-twenty meals daily or at mealtime is hard and is even more exhausting when you have to factor in the nutrition values of every meal because of the keto diet.

Keto meal planning is the way to solve the problem of cooking time, which can be hard to come by during the week, and will ensure that you eat the correct nutrients. More importantly, it is a flexible process that is owned by everyone in his or her own way so that one's needs, preferences, and schedule are conveniently accommodated.

Why You Need a Keto Meal Prep Plan

You well know that a keto diet requires certain amounts of nutrients, mainly carbohydrates, fat, and proteins per meal. Without proper planning, you can never eat right if you are on keto. Therefore, meal prepping ensures that you reach and maintain your dietary goals throughout the week by preventing you from making bad choices during the week.

Remember, for every meal you eat on a keto diet, you need a calorie breakdown as of 5% carbs, 75% fat, and 20% protein. How can you possibly achieve or ensure this every time without effective planning? Keto meal prep planning makes it possible to allocate one day to cook all the foods you will eat throughout the week and use the time you would otherwise spend cooking or thinking of what to cook on other things. A time-saver!

By doing all that planning for the whole week in one go, you reduce the stress of figuring out what to eat each day. You also save a lot of time, because you are not starting from scratch each day.

Meal prep will allow you to tailor-make meals to meet your keto needs. It is important to keep in mind that it is a process that will take time to learn but will simplify your routine if you stick to it.

Reasons for Keto Meal Prep Planning

Motivation alone is not enough for dieting or losing weight because you will never be motivated every time. There are times when your motivation will be shaken. However, researchers have found that planning is a better factor for dieting and weight-loss success.

Ninety-one percent of participants who planned

and scheduled to work out did so at least once a week while only 35% of the study group who did not schedule a workout managed to exercise at least once a week, according to a study carried in the *British Journal of Health Psychology*. Planning ahead helps you to get things done.

Moreover, there are other benefits to meal planning, which include the following:

- Less stress and time deciding what to eat
- Saves time and money
- Helps you achieve dieting needs

1.2 How This Book Is Organized

Now that you have a better understanding of what keto meal prep planning is and why it is important, let us have an overview of what is in this book. This chapter will give you an idea of how long it takes to prep meals, the benefits of keto meal planning, and steps to get you ready for meal planning.

Further ahead in the book, there will be chapters on how to begin meal prepping, easy steps for meal prepping in detail, simple go-to recipes and main keto recipes, how to do keto meal prepping on a budget.

Additionally, the remainder of the book covers meal prepping for weight loss and mistakes to avoid when doing keto meal prepping. You will get a bonus chapter on money-saving tips to help you when shopping and a section on measurements conversions so that you get your nutrients and ingredients right.

Every chapter has a "Quick Start Action Step" section to guide you on the immediate actions to take for keto meal prep planning.

1.3 How Long Does It Take to Meal-Prep?

To be honest and objective, the duration you take for meal prepping will depend on you and for a variety of reasons, the main one being your preferences and speed. There are other things you need to do, like shopping for the ingredients you will need for your meals. However, *generally, it takes about an hour to cook meal preps for a week.*

The best time to plan and prep your keto meals

would be a Saturday or Sunday, when most of us have a bit of a break from the rigors of work. Shopping in the afternoon is a good idea because you will not have to deal with the morning rush, keeping in mind that part of the reason why we are prepping is to reduce stress. You should be as relaxed and organized as possible with shopping.

Therefore, the best time to plan or decide the meals for the week would be Saturday morning before you go shopping. That means that you will have a designated time on Sunday to prep your dishes. The key to getting meal planning and prepping right is to pick a time that will be devoid of distraction or interruptions so that you can use the hour you have for cooking efficiently and optimally.

A distraction-free meal planning session is especially important for those who are starting out on keto meal prep planning. Once you are accustomed to the process, planning and prepping times will be reduced considerably. Find the best times that work for you.

A ketogenic diet requires prepping and planning because if you do not get the meals right, you will destabilize the body chemistry. To ease the process of keto meal prep, start with a week's meal plan, pick out the dishes you want for every one of the three meals per day. From the meals you have chosen, you will draw a detailed shopping list ahead of the shopping time so that you will spend as little time as possible buying them and have enough time for preparation.

The ketogenic diet meal prep plan is ideal for the busy person on the ketogenic diet who hardly ever has enough time to prepare his or her meals. If you leave for work early and are back home to sleep most of the week and you are on the keto diet, there is no better option to ensure that you keep on track despite your hectic schedule.

1.4 The Benefits of a Keto Diet Meal Prep Plan

- *It eliminates the temptation to eat off-diet.*

Remember that you are on a diet. The keto diet is calories- and nutrients-specific, such that if you falter, you are likely to destabilize your body chemistry and reverse the gains you have made.

Keto meal prepping eliminates the temptation to eat fast food or any other meals that are not healthy since you have your meals prepared beforehand. With meal planning and prepping, the foods you eat will meet your dietary needs because they are well thought out, planned, and prepped in advance. All you will need to do is warm the food and eat it.

- *Keto meal planning and prepping saves time.*

Meal planning and prepping will save you time all round. You save time with shopping since you have a list of everything you want early enough. You save time with cooking since the ingredients are prepared early, and you save time on deciding what to eat.

Consequently, you have more time to assign to other things, like spending time with family and friends, pursuing a hobby, or beating a deadline at work. You save a lot of time you would have spent cooking, shopping, and deciding meals.

- *Grocery shopping is made easy.*

Meal planning ensures that you know beforehand what you will require for your meals so that you do not leave out anything from your grocery shopping list or struggle to list items down at the last minute. The best way of detailing your shopping list is by sectionalizing the items into the various food categories, such as dairy, grains, fats, fruits, frozen foods, proteins, and veggies.

Always try to get a new food item each week for each category. If you bought tilapia last week for protein, get salmon this week. If you bought broccoli, get cauliflower this week. The list of items you buy must take into account the ketogenic diet nutritional requirement.

- *It makes meal decision-making easier and reduces stress.*

As many of you may know, settling on what to eat every day three times a week can be difficult and stressful. With keto meal prepping and planning, this problem will be completely eliminated because you do not have to make the decision every day—the decision about what to eat is made once for the whole week. The time you spend preparing your meals is significantly reduced because everything is planned ahead.

The stress that comes with deciding meals and keeping up with the requirements of your keto diet regime will also fizzle away with meal prepping. You will have a calmer and healthier mental predisposition and keep stress-related health problems at bay.

- *Keto meal prep planning saves money.*

Buying food items for your cooking in bulk saves you a lot of money. No impulse buying, no cases of buying the wrong ingredients because you will know exactly what to buy in advance. Pricing food items ahead brings in the effective element of cost control through portion control. You save money because you will not be eating out every time and will be buying items at a bargain.

Additionally, you will know the right quantities to buy, which will save you from the financial losses incurred through wastes, especially when you buy more than you need and have to throw away what is left or watch it go bad. You also save money by making fewer trips to the shop.

- *It gives you total control of what you eat and the calorie intake.*

Advance food planning and preparation gives you total control of your keto diet, enabling the consumption of the right calories and keto macros balance. The chances of you eating foods that are not recommended or going above the recommended calories are closely managed or eliminated.

You know too well that controlling what you eat, the portion, and your calorie intake is important for dieting and weight loss. Keto meal prepping will keep you within the right measures and will help you to attain ketosis for a healthy, efficient body.

- *It helps with hunger management.*

    Hunger pangs are mainly triggered by predetermined mealtimes by habit. When the time comes when you normally eat dinner, you are likely to feel hungry. Keto meal prepping and planning will help you manage hunger by ensuring that you have the dish ready for the respective meal. Eating at the right time is also important to maintain the right ketosis metabolic balance.

- *You get time to do other things.*

Whether you want to call it multitasking or getting time for other things, keto meal prepping will get that for you. The many hours you have from not cooking and preparing meals can be used for other activities, which will improve your performance and productivity in other areas of your life.

This is the ideal option for those with a busy life and an in tray that is always full. You want a meal plan in the first place because of the time factor. You are busy and would prefer getting more done within the often short time that is available to you.

Even with the meal prepping process, you will be able to have multiple meals cooking because as something is baking in the oven, you could have another dish simmering on one burner, another stew on a different burner, and another burner frying another keto recipe, all within the prep time!

- *It will bring variety to your meals.*

    Keto meal prepping ensures that you have a variety of healthy foods every weekly cycle. By alternating products within every food category, you cannot get bored with what you eat because of the variety at your disposal. As we said under the point of grocery shopping, you can eat different vegetables every day of the week or for every meal.

- *It will help you to lose weight.*

    Planning ketogenic meals in advance is key to weight loss. You will have the portions right, and the calorie intake will be as recommended. Consistency with the meals will help you to lose weight quickly.

Accordingly, this book is a great resource for those who are still looking into the keto diet and are considering whether it is the right diet for them to take up. You have the chance to learn about how keto meal prepping and planning works and how convenient it makes the dieting process for you.

Moreover, with all the benefits listed above, you will save time and money while still leading a healthy lifestyle and not compromising on your profession. In fact, you will have more time for your work and a healthy body to see you through the rigors of work.

For those on the keto diet and are not meal prepping and planning, this is another layer to the benefits you are already enjoying from the diet.

1.5 An Overview of Steps to Get Ready for Keto Meal Prepping

Now that you know the benefits of a keto meal prep plan, we will have an overview of the steps and what you need to get ready for meal prepping. As much as there may be nuances in prepping the different meals, the general structure of getting ready for food prepping will remain the same throughout.

Here is what you need to do:

- **Step 1: Decide what to eat.**

  Pick a day of the week when you have enough time to outline a meal plan for the whole week.

  Decide your meals by doing the following:

  - Evaluate what you want to eat each day of the coming week for breakfast, lunch, and supper. Include snacks or desserts as you may want.

  - Slot your picks in a calendar to correspond to the days and mealtimes.

  - Go for ready recipes that have calories indicated and, if possible, macros listed so that you can easily adapt them to your preferences.

- Account for the number of people who will be served.
- Make it simple, having one meal more than once, either cooked or as a leftover.
- Print or write down the recipe for each meal and the ingredients as required.

- **Step 2: Map and plan the meals you have chosen.**

The next thing after picking out the meals you want for a week is to map out and plan the meals to meet keto nutritional requirements. Create different nutrition combinations for fat, carbohydrates, proteins, and vegetables. These combinations will help you with portioning the meals and drawing a supporting list of things to shop for.

- **Step 3: Make a shopping list, pick a shopping day, and shop for the ingredients.**

Write down the ingredients and other requirements, pick a convenient day to buy the items on your shopping list, and then shop for the items.

- **Step 4: Cook the keto meals.**

    This is the final step in the prepping process. Once you have the ingredients ready, it is time to prep the meals and cook them accordingly.

Quick Start Action Step

For your meal prepping, follow the four steps above to cover all bases. Decide the keto diet meals you want and get the recipes, map and plan the individual meals, do a detailed shopping list and buy the required ingredients, and finally prep the ingredients and cook the meals.

Chapter 2
How to Begin Meal Prepping

FRUITS
Let fruits jazz up your feast!

- ☐ Apples
- ☐ Avocado
- ☐ Bananas
- ☐ Blueberries
- ☐ Cranberries
- ☐ Grapefruit

Chapter 2: How to Begin Meal Prepping

In this chapter, we shall look at the things you need to have ready to begin meal prepping. We shall discuss the must-have kitchen equipment for meal prepping. We shall also look at how to stock your pantry with keto essentials and the type of storage containers you need for storing the meals you prepare.

2.1 Getting Ready for Keto Meal Prepping

When you have everything in place for meal prepping—the basic kitchen utensils and equipment, the meal prepping ingredients, and storage containers—you make meal prepping much easier. Preparing the pantry staples and kitchen equipment may seem time-consuming, but the opposite is true. It will save you time for the days and weeks to come.

Before you begin meal prepping, it would be wise to know the different ways of prepping meals, which will help with saving you time on the process so that you do not end up spending a whole day prepping your week's meals. The most popular ways to meal-prep include the following:

- Individual portions: Cooking fresh meals and portioning them into individual grab-and-go meals. Refrigerate and eat over the next few days. This is best for lunches.
- Ready-to-cook meals: This involves prepping ingredients for different meals in advance to save time when cooking.
- Cooking full meals in advance: You cook all the meals you want and refrigerate them. Warm them at mealtimes. This is convenient for dinners.
- Batch cooking: Cooking a large portion of one recipe and then dividing it into several portions, freezing them, and eating them for weeks or months. Best for lunches and dinners.

The method you choose for prepping your meals will be your preference and will probably be determined by your schedule and time management goals. Mixing different meal-prepping methods can also work depending on your unique circumstances.

2.2 The Benefits of Having Essentials Ready for Meal Prepping

Meal prepping can be challenging if you are a beginner, and you should, therefore, not be surprised nor discouraged. It is very easy to get caught up in the nitty gritty in trying to get it right. However, once you have the basics learned, you should take it easy and be practical. Do not try to do everything at once, and do not seek perfection. You should allow yourself room to wriggle and make mistakes from which you will learn from as time goes by.

Prepping meals is important for getting the keto diet right. Planning and prepping your meals ahead of time will help you stay within the recommended portions and nutritional counts.

Additionally, having the essentials of meal prepping ready—the equipment, ingredients, containers, and other requirements—may save you time in prepping and cooking. You will be stress-free and will get more done faster if you have things ready, having your meals for the week ready in no time and leaving the rest of the day to rest.

2.3 The Essentials and Requirements for Meal Prepping

There are a number of kitchen equipment and tools that you must have to begin meal prepping. Additionally, you must have the essential ingredients for your recipes ready, as well as certain must-have keto diet ingredients. Having these kitchen tools and keto pantry staples is a time-saver.

The lists below have the essentials you should have ready for successful and stress-free meal prepping:

Kitchen Equipment and Tools

The following are some of the basic kitchen equipment and tools you need for prepping your keto-friendly meals. There are many household stores where you can get what you want at very affordable prices, as well as bargain sites.

a. Skillet

A cast iron skillet is a must-have in your kitchen for easy meal prepping, and it lasts a long time. It is easy to clean and offers better service than a pan. These are easy to clean and safer than using a cheap Teflon-covered pan. Plus, it helps keep your iron levels up.

b. Chef's knife

Since you will be doing a lot of dicing and slicing, you need a dependable knife that will serve you well for a long time. Getting a high-quality chef's knife will make cutting and slicing very easy.

c. Blender or food processor

The keto diet is full of meals and recipes that will require a blender or food processor. Certainly, for keto smoothies, salad dressings, homemade nut butter, etc., you will need one. A blender and processor in one is a good option instead of having two.

d. Instant Pot or pressure cooker or slow cooker

   This is the perfect kitchen essential for slow and long cooking. Some of the keto recipes you will encounter will need you to cook broths and soups or slow cook meats, which require you to have a slow cooker. You will have other parts of a recipe slow cooking as you prep others.

e. Nonstick baking paper

   Your keto oven meals and bakes will require nonstick oven paper.

f. Kitchen scale

   You will need a kitchen scale to weigh some foods and ingredients. This is a perfect product for keto diet meal prep beginners who are just learning how to stay in ketosis.

There are so many kitchen tools that you can have to make your work easier in the kitchen. Here, we have only listed what we think are the essentials for you to have for keto meal prepping.

Stocking the Pantry with the Essentials

For the pantry, there are general cooking ingredients that you must have, and then there are keto essential ingredients that you will need to stock so that you do not miss a recipe item or make several time-wasting trips to the shop.

The following are what you should have for keto meal prepping:

1. Almond flour
2. Avocado oil
3. baking powder and baking soda
4. Butter (preferably grass-fed)
5. Celery salt
6. Cheese(s)
7. Cream cheese
8. Cinnamon
9. Cocoa powder
10. Coconut aminos
11. Coconut flour
12. Coconut oil
13. Eggs (free range and pastured recommended)
14. full-fat coconut milk

15. Garlic cloves
16. Garlic powder
17. Ground beef (grass-fed recommended)
18. Heavy cream
19. Hot sauce
20. Keto sweeteners (erythritol, monk fruit, stevia, Swerve, Truvia)
21. Mayonnaise
22. MCT oil powder
23. Mustard (Dijon or yellow)
24. Nuts and seeds
25. Nut butters
26. Olive oil
27. Oregano
28. Parsley
29. Pumpkin pie spice
30. Red pepper flakes
31. Red wine vinegar
32. Sugar-free spices
33. Salt and pepper
34. Sour cream
35. Thyme
36. Unsweetened yogurt
37. Vanilla extract

38. high-fat oils

These are simply the essentials. You may stock as many as you want as long as they fit in the keto diet.

2.4 Storage Containers to Use

The containers you choose for storing your food storage can turn your food from a fabulous meal to an unenjoyable dish. Glass containers are the best for food storage because they are safe for microwave heating and warming. They do not have harmful chemicals as found in plastics.

In fact, use only glass containers for keto meal prepping, and make sure they are made for the microwave and oven.

Recommended Food Storage Container Specifications

- Airtight—to keep food fresh.
- BPA-free microwavable containers—go for Pyrex glassware.

- Compartmentalized containers—to enable you to have the different parts of a meal in one container.
- Freezer-safe containers—to limit freezer burn.
- Leak-proof
- Stackable—for better space management.

There are a lot of container options on the market for you to pick from. As long as they can be used in the oven or the microwave to heat or warm your food and they meet the recommended food storage specifications above, the glass container will be good for use. You should also get them in different sizes so that you can pack different portions and recipes conveniently.

A high-quality food storage container should ensure that the nutrients in the food do not deteriorate quickly and that the food stays fresh and retains its taste.

Quick Start Action Step

Now that you know the basics required of you to have before meal prepping, if you are a beginner, we would recommend shopping for the items you do not have a day before the actual meal prep, preferably when you will be shopping for recipe ingredients.

Meal planning and prepping is best on weekends, when you are likely to have sufficient time to do it without distractions and disruptions. Saturday for shopping and Sunday for prepping works well.

Chapter 3
Easy Steps to Meal Prepping

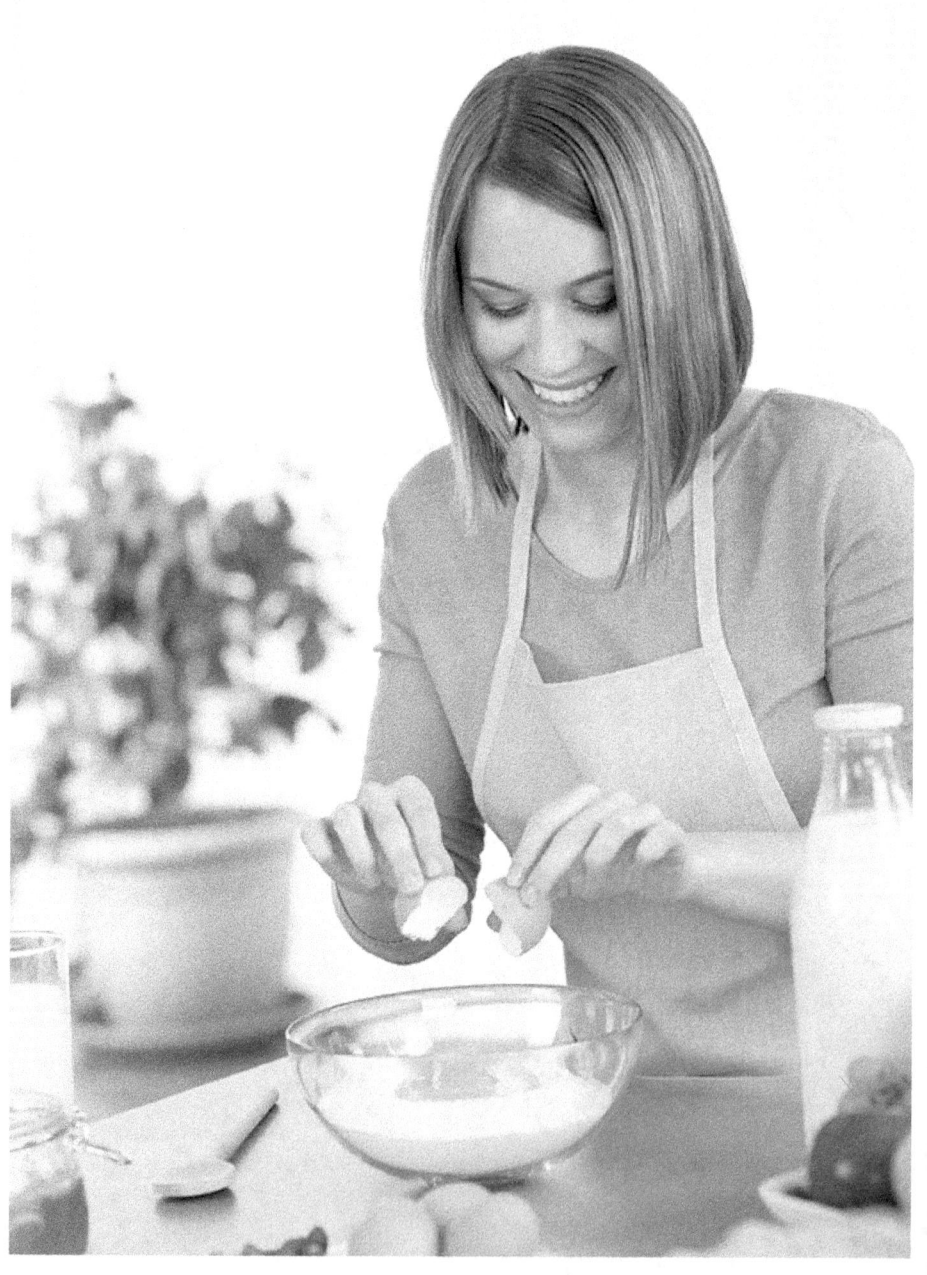

Chapter 3: Easy Steps to Meal Prepping

This chapter will outline easy steps to guide you through successful keto meal prepping from beginning to end. You will mention the benefits of going by these steps and discuss each step of keto meal prepping in detail. Additionally, we will give you insights on how to calculate macros and why that is important.

3.1 How to Calculate Macros

We already know that for you to be successful with ketogenic dieting, you must plan every step and ensure that everything is done right. Calculating macros is one of the important aspects of ensuring success if you are on a keto diet.

To eat right, you need to pick the right keto recipes, which will require you to look at the calorie and macro contents of each meal and each day. Macros are the three main macronutrients of the keto diet, namely, fat, protein, and carbohydrates. While a regular diet is heavily reliant on carbs, the keto diet is fat-oriented.

You will need to eat foods with high quantities of fat, moderate protein, and very little carbs. It is easy when said; however, getting it right with every meal needs a keen tracking of the macro content. Every meal you eat on keto meal plan should be 75% fat, 20% protein, and 5% total carbohydrates.

For instance, if you are on 2,000 calories per day, the breakdown will be as follows:

- 1,500 calories or 167 grams of fat

- 400 calories or 100 grams of protein

- 100 calories or 25 grams of carbs

To achieve and maintain ketosis, you will have to make sure that your nutrients per meal are maintained at the quantities broken down above and have carbs at 25 grams or below.

For beginners, making macro calculation is a must. The good news is that the longer you stay on the diet, the easier it will get, and you will easily know your ratios depending on the recipe once you are familiar with the meals.

To calculate macros effectively, you will need a ketogenic calculator which will give you calculations for a classic ketogenic diet (75% fat, 20% protein, 5% carbohydrate), which is the recommended keto diet and a specialized macro calculation function for more specificity in calculation of macros where you can input specific figures for fat, protein, and carbohydrate.

How to Use the Ketogenic Macro Calculator

Here is how the calculator works:

- **Step 1: Pick the macro calculating option—standard or specialized.**

    You pick between the standard ketogenic diet calculator and the specialized macronutrient calculator. Beginners and those on the classic keto diet should work with the standard option, which is straightforward and is easy to use. It works on the basis of the standard percentages of carbs, fats, and protein in the normal keto diet.

    The second option, specialized macro calculator, computes specific carb and protein targets, which you choose, thus not based on the classic keto ratios. There are several reasons why some people would want to do this.

It is important to note that this function is best left to those who have been on keto for some time, have achieved ketosis, and have a good understanding of how the diet works for them and interacts with their bodies.

When to use the standard keto calculation option:

- If you do not know your ketosis macros ratios.

- If you want exact ratios for every meal.

- If you are new to the ketogenic diet.

- If your reason for dieting is simply to lose, gain, or maintain weight.

When to use the specialized macronutrient calculation option:

- Pregnant or breastfeeding women who are measuring macros based on doctor advice.

- If you are adjusting macros ratios because of the keto rash.

- If your doctor recommends different macros ratios from the standard.

- If you know the exact grams of carbs and protein macros to aim for.

- If you have specific macro needs, e.g., an athlete.

- If you are on a high-protein keto diet.

The specialized macronutrient calculator should be used by those on keto who have special macros needs because of issues, like a very active lifestyle (athlete), a medical condition, or pregnancy.

- **Step 2: Enter the basal metabolic rate (BMR) details.**

The next step is to add your basic details. The calculator needs information about your age, gender, height, and weight to come up with your basal metabolic rate (BMR)—the amount of energy your body spends, per unit, while at rest.

How your bio details affect Your BMR:

- o Age: BMR shrinks with age, starting after about thirty years, because of muscle mass decline.

- o Gender: The body composition and performance of female and male differ.

- o Height and weight: Needed to compute your unique body composition.

- **Step 3: Input how active you are.**

Next, the calculator needs to factor in how active you are. Physical activity level (PAL) determines how much energy you burn daily when active. Your BMR outcome and PAL will be combined to calculate your total daily energy expenditure (TDEE)—the number of calories your body burns daily. This will then decide the daily calorie content to compensate what you burn.

- **Step 4: Set dieting goals.**

This is the point when you tell the calculator why you are on the keto diet. What results are you working toward? You state whether you want to maintain, gain, or lose weight, inputting a calorie deficit, surplus, or a zero depending on what you want to achieve.

For example:

Choosing 20% calories deficit reduces your daily calories by 20% of what you actually need, thus resulting in moderate weight loss.

- **Step 5: Use the specialized calculator's advanced fields—body fat percentage, protein ratio, and total carb intake.**

This is the step in the specialized calculator option that factors in specific macro ratios as entered. The body fat percentage, protein ratio, and carbs intake are considered. *Body fat percentage*, which determines lean body mass, enables calculation of a more accurate TDEE. Subsequently, the protein ratio you require per day for weight loss without losing muscle is arrived at.

3.2 The Benefits of Following These Steps for Keto Goals

The benefits of keto meal prep planning are probably what has got you interested in the keto diet in the first place or what led you to pick this book. The benefits of the steps here are the overall keto meal prepping and planning benefits as discussed in detail earlier in chapter 1. Here is a quick recap of the advantages following these steps for meal prepping before we discuss the steps in detail.

The following is a list of the benefits of keto meal prep planning:

1. It saves time as compared to cooking daily.

2. Meal prepping is cheaper than cooking every day.

3. You do not decide what to eat every day.

4. You have better control your food portions.

5. You have better calorie and macro management.

6. Homemade food, especially by yourself, is delicious, healthier, and safer.

7. You have everything ready for cooking ahead of time.

3.3 Keto Meal Prep Planning Steps

1. *Plan the Meal Prep*

Planning entails picking a day for keto meal prepping, picking the meals you want for the week, and settling on the right recipes for the meals.

- *Pick the prepping day.*

    The first thing to do is to pick the day for prepping the meals. Sunday is the best day because most people are off work and can enlist the help of others if you want. Some people opt for two days in a week to prep, which allows them to split meal prepping into two, usually Sunday and Wednesday.

- *Choose the meals.*

Once you have a day or have decided to split meal prepping into two days, choose the meals you want. Since we are focused on planning for a whole week, choose all the meals, desserts, and snack that you want. Ensure that the meals are healthy and are keto compliant. You can also mark the meals on a calendar at this point.

- *Pick meal recipes.*

Once you know the meals you want, the next thing to do is to find keto recipes for the meals you have chosen. Keep the calories and macros in mind when picking the recipes so that you balance the meals correctly.

Beginners should choose easy recipes with a few ingredients. Even better, go for recipes that have similar ingredients—for instance, different meals with meats or vegetables—to make shopping and cooking easier.

Knowledge of how macronutrients are converted into calories will help you keep the right ratios. When choosing recipes, select the ones that you want to eat and will enjoy. It should not just be healthy, you should be happy about it.

- *Write down the week's keto menu.*

Once you have the recipes, write them down in the order you want to eat them during the week. Write down or print out the recipes so that you have them to follow on prep day. It also helps to craft the order in which the food is prepared. Start with the more engaging meals and finish up with the easy ones, like those for breakfast, desserts, and snacks.

- *Pick a prep day.*

This is the point where you decide if you want to do it on Saturday or Sunday or if you want to prep twice, say on Wednesday and Sunday. As advised earlier, it works best to prep a day after shopping, or you can choose to prep the same day you shop.

2. Write Down the Shopping List

Draw a shopping list of the ingredients from each of the recipes you have settled on. Break down the list into food categories—dairy, meat, vegetables, etc. The list must have the exact quantities of each ingredient as per the keto recipes. Avoid packaged and processed products.

Tip: Always check your fridge, freezer, and pantry to confirm what you have so that you do not overstock.

3. Go Shopping for the Items You Listed

Once you have the shopping list, all you have left is to buy what you need before you embark on the actual prepping. As said earlier, pick a convenient shopping day and time so that you are not drained by the experience. Shop when there is less traffic in the shops so that you will easily get what you want to leave.

Apart from the recipe items, buy the keto pantry essentials we listed earlier—any kitchen equipment and storage containers enough for the meals you will be preparing. Make sure you have your shopping list and stick to buying the items in it as planned.

4. Cook and Store the Meals

This is the point you have been preparing for—making the effort count and turning the recipes into delicious meals. Have all ingredients ready and the recipes out when doing this and follow them step by step.

Cooking can be tricky and may take longer than planned or suggested by the respective recipes, but keep going. It will be easier as you go along. Read through the recipes to understand what you need to do and how to do it. It is a good idea to start with those meals with the longest preparation process.

Those that need to be marinated or simmered for long periods should be dealt with first before the cooking day or hour so that everything is ready for the finalization of the dishes. All the veggies and meats that need to be prepared (cutting, slicing, dicing, marinating, etc.) should be done earlier so that they are ready on your cooking day. You may want to do this on shopping day after making your purchases or very early in the morning on prep day.

When packing the foods for storage, take into account the storage life of the various constituents of the meals packed, as well as recommended refrigeration times after cooking. For example, cut vegetables, like onions and peppers, will stay fresh under refrigeration for up to three days. Leafy vegetable if dried will last about a week, and cooked grains and meat dishes should be eaten within four days of cooking. Warm the meals at respective healthy temperatures when eating.

Tips:

- Newbies to keto and to meal prep should begin small and gradually prepare more meals once they learn and identify their favorite recipes and get a handle on meal prepping respectively.

- When you start, choose simple recipes with a few ingredients and pick recipes with similar ingredients to shorten your shopping list and make cooking faster.

- If you are a beginner, you do not have to do a whole week. Try preparing three meals for starters to have a feel of the process.

- Start with some recipes that you have prepared before.

- Plan meals around seasonal produce for freshness and price value.

- Preparing the same dish for two or three mealtimes is a good energy-saving and time-saving idea for beginners.

Quick Start Action Step

Meal prepping is not a complicated process, is it? It may seem like at first, especially for a beginner when you move from reading to actual doing.

Now what you need to do is to act on the steps learned here and follow through on the keto meal prep planning. Pick the meals you want and decide the meal prep day. Draw your shopping list to cover the ingredients, buy everything you need, and finally cook your meals and store them for the week ahead.

There is no better satisfaction than eating a delicious healthy meal prepared by yourself.

Chapter 4
Simple Go-To Recipes to Start

Chapter 4: Simple Go-To Recipes to Start

Meal prepping is not as it seems for beginners. In fact, it can be overwhelming since you have to pick out recipes fit for a diet that you have just started following, then prepare several meals on this new dieting regime. Find here simple, easy-to-fix go-to recipes to make on a weekend that you can start with.

Some of the benefits of using the recipes shared here for beginners:

- Time-saving
- Easy to prepare and short cooking times
- Ketogenic compliant
- Avoid the stress of identifying meals
- Money-saving

4.1 The Recipes

Here are simple keto recipes for beginners:

Breakfast Recipes

1. Bacon-and-Egg Muffins (Cups)

Bacon-and-eggs muffins are a quick low-carb breakfast fix for breakfast and will give your body an infusion of energy and protein. It is high in fat, which is perfect for the keto diet. Once you have everything baking in the oven, you can work on with other things as you wait for the oven ringer. Use gluten- and nitrate-free bacon.

Prep: 5 minutes

Cook: 35 minutes

Total: 40 minutes

Calories (350), fat (26 g), carbs (1 g), protein (26 g)

Ingredients

- 12 slices sugar-free bacon

- 8 eggs

- 1/2 cup shredded cheddar cheese

- a pinch of salt

- 1/4 teaspoon black pepper

- 1/4 cup diced green onions/scallions

- 1/2 cup chopped fresh spinach

Instructions

1. Preheat oven to 350°F.

2. Put the cheese, eggs, pepper, and salt together and whip with a fork.

3. Prepare 12 muffin tins. Spray them with nonstick cooking oil.

4. Place the bacon strips inside each muffin cup on the sides.

5. Fill each muffin cup with the cheese, eggs, pepper, and salt mixture, 3/4 full, ensuring that it is surrounded by the bacon strip.

6. Sprinkle scallions on top of the mixture in the muffin cup.

7. Bake until the egg cups are golden brown, 30–35 minutes.

8. Once baked, scoop them out of the tins with a knife.

9. Serve.

Tip

If prepping the muffins ahead of time, let it cool for 10 minutes after baking, wrap each in saran wrap, and then freeze in a freezer Ziploc. Thaw overnight in fridge and microwave for up to 1 minute to eat.

2. Fried Eggs and Avocado

Prep: 5 minutes

Cook: 8 minutes

Total: 13 minutes

Fat (24.1 g), carbs (12.4 g), protein (13 g)

Ingredients

- 2 eggs

- 1/2 avocado (peeled, pitted, and cubed)

- 1 tablespoon butter

- salt and pepper to taste

Instructions

1. Heat skillet on medium-high heat.

2. Melt butter in skillet.

3. Place eggs into the skillet on one side and place avocado pieces on the other.

4. Stir avocados.

5. Flip eggs after four minutes.

6. Continue to cook eggs for another four minutes.

7. Once eggs are cooked, place them on a plate.

8. Scoop avocado over eggs, and season with salt and pepper if desired.

3. Sausage Patty Avocado Cheese Sandwich

Prep: 5 minutes

Total time: 5 minutes

Protein (22 g), fat (54 g), carbs (7 g)

Ingredients

- 2 sausage patties

- 1 egg

- 1 tablespoon cream cheese

- 1 teaspoon sharp cheddar

- sliced medium avocado

- 1/4–1/2 teaspoon sriracha (to taste)

- salt and pepper to taste

Instructions

- Fry sausages in a skillet over medium heat.

- Melt cream cheese and sharp cheddar in a small bowl.

- Mix cheese and sriracha.

- Season eggs and do an omelet.

- Fill the omelet with cheese and sriracha mixture.

- Complete sandwich.

Snack and Side Recipes

1. Sheet Pan Garlic Parmesan Roasted Broccoli and Green Beans

Prep: 5 minutes

Cook: 20 minutes

Total time: 25 minutes

Ingredients

- 2 heads of broccoli

- broccoli stems, cut into pieces

- 350 grams green beans

- 1 cup grape or cherry tomatoes

- 1/3 cup freshly grated Parmesan cheese
- 1/4 cup olive oil
- half a lemon's juice
- 1 tablespoon minced garlic
- salt and pepper

Instructions

- Preheat the oven to 200°C (400°F).
- Spray nonstick oil on baking sheet or tray.
- Place broccoli and green beans tray.
- Sprinkle Parmesan cheese.
- Sprinkle olive oil and lemon juice.

- Add minced garlic and salt and pepper to season.

- Mix until all the vegetables are covered in dressing.

- Place in oven and bake for 20 minutes.

- Remove sheet and add the tomatoes to the pan after 20 minutes.

- Flip vegetables and put back in the oven to cook evenly.

- Bake for another 5–20 minutes until cooked through. The broccoli florets should be crisp.

- Top with the remaining Parmesan cheese.

2. Kale Chips

Calories (98), fat (7 g), saturated fat (1 g), carbs (6 g), fiber (1 g), protein (3 g)

Ingredients

- 2 large stalks kale
- 1 tablespoon avocado oil
- 1 1/2 tablespoon TBS nutritional yeast
- 1/2 teaspoon garlic powder
- 1/4 teaspoon cumin
- 1/4 teaspoon chili powder
- 1/8 teaspoon cayenne
- 1/4 teaspoon pink salt

Instructions

- Preheat oven to 300°F.

- Oil a large baking sheet.

- Separate kale leaves from the stalk.

- Dry the kale leaves.

- Place the kale leaves in a bowl and sprinkle with 1/2 tablespoon avocado oil.

- Massage oil into the kale leaves with your fingers.

- Sprinkle 1 tablespoon nutritional yeast.

- Add 1/2 tablespoon of yeast.

- Set the leaves to the oiled baking sheet and sprinkle remaining nutritional yeast.

- Bake kale at 300°F for 7–9 minutes

- Watching closely for the right crispy texture.

3. Paleo Scotch Eggs

Prep: 10 minutes

Cook: 30 minutes

Total: 40 minutes

Calories (169), fat (8.2 g), carbohydrates (0.67 g), sugars (0.49 g), protein (23.1 g)

Ingredients

- eggs
- 500 grams (1 pound) minced pork or another meat
- 2 teaspoon herb or spice
- 1/2 teaspoon salt

Instructions

- Boil eggs for 4 minutes.
- Remove eggs and dip in cold water.
- Peel the eggs and dry with paper towel.
- Mix the minced meat with spices.
- Flatten a handful of minced meat like a patty.
- Place the egg patty and cover the egg with the meat.
- Place on an oiled baking tray.
- Bake for 30 minutes at 180°C (350°F).

Lunch Recipes

1. Mexican Turkey Burgers

Prep: 15 minutes

Cook: 15 minutes

Carbs (0.3 g), fat (34.5 g), protein (16.8 g), calories (380)

Ingredients

- 1 pound ground turkey

- 1/3 cup finely chopped red bell pepper

- finely chopped cilantro-1/4 cup

- finely sliced green onions-2

- 2 cloves grated or finely minced garlic

- 1/2 lime, 1 tablespoon juice

- 1/2 teaspoon salt

- 1 tablespoon olive oil

Instructions

- Preheat grill medium to high heat.

- Mix ground turkey, red bell pepper, cilantro, green onions, garlic, lime juice, and salt in a bowl.

- Mix it with a fork.

- Flatten into 4 patties.

- Sprinkle the patties with olive oil and salt.

- Grill the burger patties for 5–8 minutes each side until internal temperature is 165 °F.

2. Cheeseburger Lettuce Wraps

Prep: 15 minutes

Cook: 8 minutes

Carbs (0.3 g), fat (34.5 g), protein (16.8 g), calories (380)

Ingredients

- 2 pounds lean ground beef
- ½ teaspoon seasoned salt
- 1 teaspoon black pepper
- 1 teaspoon dried oregano
- 6 slices American cheese
- 2 large heads iceberg or romaine lettuce, rinsed and dry
- 2 thinly sliced tomatoes
- thinly sliced small red onion

Spread:

- 1/4 cup light mayo

- 3 tablespoons ketchup

- 1 tablespoon dill pickle relish

- salt and pepper

Instructions

- On medium, heat a grill or skillet.

- Mix ground beef, seasoned salt, pepper, and oregano in a large bowl.

- Divide into 6 then roll into balls.

- Flatten each ball into a patty.

- Grill patties for about 4 minutes on each side or until cooked.

- Add cheese to each cooked patty.

- Place each patty on a large piece of lettuce.

- Smear spread.

- Wrap patties with lettuce.

3. *Avocado Tuna Salad Recipe*

Calories (304), fat (20 g), carbohydrates (9 g), protein (22 g)

Ingredients

- 15 ounces (3 small cans) tuna in oil, drained and flaked

- 1 English cucumber, sliced

- 2 large medium avocados (peeled, pitted, and sliced)

- 1 small/medium red onion, thinly sliced

- 1/4 cup cilantro

- 2 tablespoons lemon juice freshly squeezed

- 2 tablespoons extra-virgin olive oil

- 1 teaspoon sea salt to taste

- 1/8 teaspoon black pepper

Instructions

- Mix sliced cucumber, sliced avocado, thinly sliced red onion, drained tuna, and 1/4 cup cilantro in a large bowl.

- Sprinkle the mixture with 2 tablespoons of lemon juice, 2 tablespoons of olive oil, 1 teaspoon of salt, and 1/8 teaspoon black pepper.

Dinner Recipes

1. *Spicy Mustard Thyme Chicken and Coconut Roasted Brussels Sprouts*

Carbs (0.3 g), fat (34.5 g), protein (16.8 g), calories (380)

Prep: 10 minutes

Cook: 25 minutes

Ingredients

- 1 pound Brussels sprouts, half sliced

- 2 medium chicken breasts, skinless and boneless

- 1/4 cup ground spicy mustard

- 1 tablespoon lemon juice

- 1 teaspoon thyme

- salt and pepper

- 1 tablespoon melted coconut oil

Instructions

- Whisk the spicy mustard, lemon juice, salt, pepper, and thyme.

- Dip chicken breasts and cover with mustard.

- Marinate for 10 minutes in the refrigerator then move to room temperature for 15 minutes before cooking.

- Preheat oven to 350 F.

- Prepare a nonstick oven paper.

- Place Brussels sprouts in a bowl and mix with melted coconut oil, salt, and pepper.

- Place Brussels sprouts on baking sheets.

- Put marinated chicken in a glass baking pan.

- Bake chicken in the oven at 350°F for 10 minutes.

- After 10 minutes, put the Brussels sprouts in the oven and bake both for 15 minutes.

2. Fathead Pizza

Calories: 110 kcal

Prep: 10 minutes

Cook: 10 minutes

Total: 20 minutes

Carbs (0.3 g), fat (34.5 g), protein (16.8 g), calories (380)

Ingredients

- 1 1/2 cups shredded mozzarella cheese
- 2 tablespoons cubed cream cheese
- 2 beaten eggs
- 1/3 cup coconut flour

Instructions

- Preheat the oven to 425°F (218°C) and then line a baking sheet or pizza pan with baking paper.
- Mix cubed cream cheese and shredded mozzarella in a bowl.

- Warm in a microwave for 90 seconds then stir at 45 seconds. Stir again after the 90 seconds until consistently mixed.

- Mix in the eggs and coconut flour.

- Knead into a dough forms. Microwave dough for 10–15 seconds to soften it if it hardens before it is well mixed.

- Spread the dough on a baking-paper-lined baking pan to about 1/4 or 1/3 inches thick.

- Poke holes with a toothpick or fork on the crust.

- Bake for 6 minutes.

- Poke more holes in any places with bubbles forming.

- Bake for an additional 3–7 more minutes until it turns golden brown.

3. Pan Lemon Chicken with Asparagus

Prep: 5 minutes

Cook: 25 minutes

Total: 30 minutes

Calories (298), fat (11 g), carbohydrates (13 g), protein (35 g)

Pan lemon chicken with braised asparagus in lemon mustard sauce is a healthy meal. It is also easy to prepare and is packed with keto nutrients.

Ingredients

- 4 skinless chicken breasts boneless

- 1/4 cup plain gluten-free flour or tapioca flour for paleo

- 2 tablespoons olive oil

- 3/4 teaspoon sea salt plus more for seasoning

- 1/2 teaspoon ground black pepper

- ground black pepper for seasoning

- 1 pound asparagus stalks, trim and cut in half

- 2 cloves crushed garlic

- 3 tablespoons fresh lemon juice

- zest of 1/2 lemon

- 1 tablespoon Dijon mustard

- 1 cup chicken stock, buy low-sodium stock

- 1 tablespoon fresh parsley, roughly chopped

- parsley for garnishing

Instructions

- Pound the chicken breasts between two plastic cling wraps, evenly thick. It will enable the chicken to cook evenly and make it more tender. If the chicken breasts are too thick, slice them lengthwise in half.

- Coat the breasts in the flour, salt, and pepper in a dish or bowl. Mix well until completely covered.

- Add 1 tablespoon of olive oil in a large skillet and heat on medium-high heat.

Add the chicken to the skillet and cook each side for about 5 minutes or until golden brown once the oil is hot. Make sure it is cooked through.

- Remove the chicken and set on a serviette-lined plate once cooked.

- In the remaining 1 tablespoon of olive oil, sauté the asparagus stalks in the skillet for one minute. Add garlic and sauté for another minute until it gives an aroma.

- In a small bowl or cup, whisk together the lemon juice and mustard until fully mixed. Pour into the skillet with the asparagus along with the chicken stock and the zest. Bring the liquid to a boil and then reduce down to a simmer. Cover and let it cook for another 3–4 minutes or until the asparagus is tender.

- Stir in the parsley and then add the chicken back to the pan and rotate the breasts to coat in the liquids. Taste the sauce and season with more salt and pepper as needed.

Desserts Recipes

1. Keto Avocado Brownies

This avocado dessert is delicious and creamy. It is a great keto recipe with low-carb content, and it is made from sugar-free chocolate.

Prep: 10 minutes

Cook: 35 minutes

Total: 45 minutes

Ingredients

- 250 grams avocado (about 2)
- 1/2 teaspoon vanilla
- 4 tablespoons cocoa powder

- 1 teaspoon stevia powder or monk fruit powder
- 3 tablespoons refined coconut oil or butter, ghee, shortening, lard
- 2 eggs
- 100 grams melted Lily's chocolate chips

Dry Ingredients

- 90 grams blanched almond flour
- 1/4 teaspoon baking soda
- 1 teaspoon baking powder
- 1/4 teaspoon salt
- 60 milliliters erythritol (or xylitol)

Instructions

- Preheat the oven to 350°F (180°C).
- Blend the avocado until smooth.
- Add the ingredients one at a time until all are in, but for the dry ingredients, put them in the blender or food processor.

- Mix together the dry ingredients and whisk. Add to the food processor and mix until combined.
- Pour the blended mixture evenly on a baking tray and bake for about 35 minutes.

2. Almond Cookies

Protein (4.8 g), carbs (8.6 g), fat (23.2 g), fiber (3.5 g), calories (247)

Ingredients

- 3 tablespoons almond butter, unsweetened
- 1.5 tablespoons coconut oil
- 1/2 large egg
- 1 teaspoon vanilla extract
- 1/8 teaspoon salt
- 1 packet Stevia
- 1/2 cup unsweetened shredded coconut
- 16 almonds

- 1.5 ounces 85% dark chocolate

Instructions

- Preheat oven to 350°F.
- Mix almond butter, coconut oil, egg, vanilla, sea salt, and sweetener in a bowl until well mixed.
- Add the coconut mix in well.
- Form 8 cookies on a baking-paper-lined baking tray using a tablespoon to pour and form into balls.
- Press two almonds into the top of each cookie.
- Bake them for 10 minutes, then let cool.
- Pour molten chocolate onto the oven tray and press the cookies on the chocolate to coat the cookie base with chocolate.
- Sprinkle the remaining chocolate on top of the cookies.

3. Cheesy Bacon-Stuffed Mini Peppers

Prep: 15 minutes

Cook: 12 minutes

Total: 27 minutes

Calories (87), fat (7 g), carbohydrates (1 g), protein (2 g)

Ingredients

- half sliced mini sweet peppers, membranes and seeds removed
- 4 ounces cream cheese
- 2 tablespoons sliced green onions
- 4 slices cooked and crumbled bacon
- 1/2 teaspoon garlic powder
- 1/2 cup shredded cheddar cheese
- Extra cheese for topping
- 1 teaspoon Worcestershire sauce
- cilantro, chopped (optional)

Instructions

- Preheat oven to 400°F.
- Spray nonstick cooking spray on a cookie sheet or oven tray.
- Mix together the bacon, garlic powder, cheddar, cream cheese, green onions, and Worcestershire sauce until smooth.
- Fill the sliced peppers with the mix, a tablespoon each.
- Put on the baking sheet or oven tray and sprinkle with extra cheese.
- Bake for 10–12 minutes until the cheese melts and the peppers are soft.

Quick Start Action Step

There you have it—fifteen great simple go-to recipes for beginners or anyone who wants a quick-fix keto meal. Pick one of the meals from each section daily to start you on the keto diet if you are a newbie. It will save you time and the stress of researching recipes.

Chapter 5
The Main Recipes

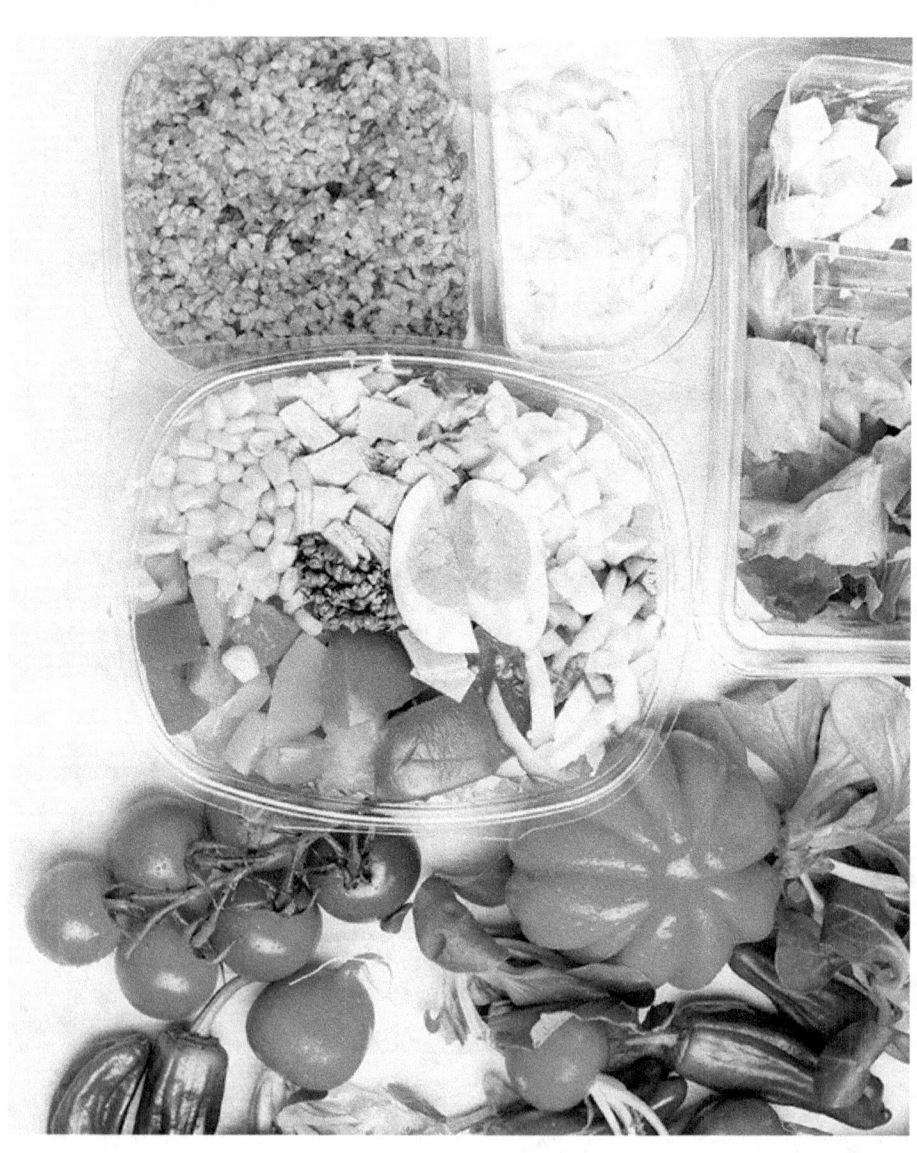

Chapter 5: The Main Recipes

This chapter will outline some of the main keto recipes that you should graduate to once you have a grasp of keto meal prepping from the simple recipes in chapter 4.

5.1 Breakfast Recipes

If you are a beginner on the keto diet, making breakfast may be the most challenging; however, it does not need to be. Preparing a keto breakfast is nothing different from how you prepare other meals. First and most important, start with the macros and then let the macros guide you to the most nutritious foods.

Here is what to do:

- Pick your protein.
- Pair with a low-carb vegetable.
- Include a healthy fat.
- Replace grains with low carb alternatives.
- Remove grains altogether.

- Change the way you make your morning beverage.

1. Ketogenic White Pizza Frittata

These are great when microwaved, reheated in the oven, or just plain cold. This recipe makes use of different cheeses in the frittata base and a top with mozzarella and pepperoni combo. Inside you find spinach that makes sure we get some greens.

The texture is a bit more on the dense side for a frittata due to the melted ricotta and Parmesan cheese inside.

Ingredients

- 12 large eggs
- 9 ounces bag of frozen spinach
- 1 ounce pepperoni
- 5 ounces mozzarella cheese
- 1 teaspoon minced garlic

- 1/2 cup fresh ricotta cheese
- 1/2 cup Parmesan cheese
- 4 tablespoons olive oil
- 1/4 teaspoon nutmeg
- salt and pepper

Instructions

- Place the frozen spinach into the microwave for between 3 and 4 minutes or until defrosted. However, it should not be hot. Squeeze the spinach using your hands and drain as much water as you can. Set it aside.
- Preheat the oven to 375°F. Mix the eggs, olive oil, and spices. Whisk well until properly mixed.
- Add in the ricotta cheese, Parmesan cheese, and spinach. Break the spinach into small pieces using your hands while adding.

- Pour the mixture into a cast iron skillet then sprinkle mozzarella cheese on the top. Add pepperoni on top of that.

- Bake it for half an hour. In case you are using a glass container in place of cast iron, bake it for 45 minutes or until it is completely set.

- Slice it up and devour it. You can top it up using crème fraîche, ranch dressing, or your favorite fatty sauce.

2. Ketogenic Brownie Muffins (6 servings)

Carbs (3.3 g), fat (13.4 g), protein (7 g), calories (183)

These breakfast muffins are rich, hearty, and moist. Far from that, they are low in carbs and high in fibers because of their flaxseed base and wholesome ingredients. Each muffin offers a rich and dark taste of chocolate with a hint of caramel. These muffins are satisfying and can keep you full until lunch hour. Furthermore, they are not hard to make.

Ingredients

- 1 cup golden flaxseed meal
- 1/4 cup cocoa powder
- 1 tablespoon cinnamon
- 1/2 tablespoon baking powder
- 1/2 teaspoon of salt
- 1 large egg
- 2 tablespoons coconut oil
- 1/4 cup sugar-free caramel syrup
- 1/2 cup pumpkin puree
- 1/2 teaspoon vanilla extract
- 1/2 teaspoon apple cider vinegar
- 1/4 cup slivered almonds

Method of Preparation

- Preheat the oven to 350°F and mix all the dry ingredients in a mixing bowl.

- In a different bowl, mix all the wet ingredients.

- Pour all the wet ingredients into the dry ingredients and mix well.

- Line a muffin tin with paper liners and spoon about 1/4 cup of batter into each liner. Sprinkle the slivered almonds over each muffin and gently press for them to stick.

- Bake in the oven for a quarter of an hour.

- Enjoy when warm or cool.

3. Ketogenic Lemon Poppy Seed Muffins (12 servings)

Carbs (1.5 g), fat (11.3 g), protein (3.7 g), calories (129)

They take less time to make and store. They contain 1.5 grams of net carbs per muffin. When fresh, their bottoms crust up well and add the extra crunch when they come out of the oven.

Ingredients

- 3/4 cup blanched almond flour
- 1/4 cup golden flaxseed meal
- 1/3 cup erythritol
- 1 tablespoon baking powder
- 2 tablespoons poppy seeds
- 1/4 cup salted butter, melted
- 1/4 cup heavy cream
- 3 large eggs
- zest of two lemons
- 3 tablespoons lemon juice
- 1 tablespoon vanilla extract
- 25 drops liquid stevia

Method of Preparation

- Preheat the oven to 350 F. In a bowl, use a fork to mix the almond flour, flaxseed meal, erythritol, and poppy seeds.

- Stir in the melted butter, eggs, and the heavy cream until smooth. Make sure that there are no lumps in the batter.

- Once it becomes smooth, add in the baking powder, liquid stevia, vanilla extract, and lemon zest and lemon juice. Mix thoroughly.

- Divide the batter equally among 12 cupcake molds.

- Bake for 20 minutes or until they slightly turn brown.

- Remove from the oven and let it cool for 10 minutes.

4. Bacon Cheddar Chive Omelet (1 serving)

Carbs (1 g), fat (39 g), protein (24 g), calories (463)

The bacon offers a burst of flavor with the eggs and cheese. The chives offer a sweet onion taste.

Ingredients

- 2 slices cooked bacon
- 1 teaspoon bacon fat
- 2 large eggs
- 1 ounce cheddar cheese
- 2 stalks chives
- salt and pepper

Method of Preparation

- Ensure that you have all the ingredients ready because the omelet cooks quite fast. Shred the cheese, precook the bacon, and chop the chives.

- Heat a pan with bacon fat in it at medium-low heat. Add the eggs then season with chives, salt, and pepper.

- As soon as the edges start to set, add the bacon to the center and let it cook for around 30 seconds longer. You then turn off the heat.

- Add the cheese on top the bacon and make sure it's centered. You then take two edges of the omelet and fold them onto the cheese. Hold the edges for a moment as the cheese partially melts to act as an adhesive to hold them in place.

- Do the same with the other edges creating a burrito of sorts. You then flip it over and let it cook for a little longer in the warm pan.

- Serve with extra cheese, bacon, and chives if you like.

5. *Ketogenic Breakfast Burger (2 servings)*

Carbs (3 g), fat (56 g), protein (30.5 g), calories (655)

This is an option for brunch or heavy breakfast.

Ingredients

- 4 ounces sausage
- 2 ounces pepper jack cheese
- 4 slices bacon
- 2 large eggs
- 1 tablespoon butter
- 1 tablespoon PB fit powder
- salt and pepper

Method of Preparation

1. Begin by cooking the bacon. Lay the strips on a wire rack over a cookie sheet. Bake at 400°F for 25 minutes or until crisp.

2. Mix together butter and PB fit powder in a small container to rehydrate. Set aside.

3. Form sausage patties and cook in a pan over medium to high heat. Turn over when the bottom side is browned.

4. Grate the cheese and have it ready.

5. As soon as the other side of the sausage patty is browned, add the cheese and cover with a lid.

6. Remove the sausage patties with the melted cheese and set aside. Fry an egg in the same pan.

7. Bring everything together—sausage patty, egg, bacon, and the rehydrated PB fit on top.

6. Chocolate Sea Salt Smoothie

This smoothie is silky and smooth and tastes great, and it is packed with good fats and ketones.

Benefits of coconut and coconut yogurt:

- Antioxidants
- Vitamins and minerals
- Lactose-free
- High fiber content
- Lauric acid

- Active and live cultures like milk-based yogurts
- Good source of bone-building calcium

Prep: 5 minutes

Cook: 0 minutes

Total time: 5 minutes

Ingredients

- 3 large egg yolks
- 1/3 unsweetened coconut yogurt
- 1 tablespoon tahini
- 1/4 cup cocoa powder
- 20 drops stevia
- 2 scoops Exogenous Ketone Base, chocolate flavored
- 12 ounces water

Instructions

- Mix all the ingredients and blend until smooth.

7. Turkey Sausage Frittata

Frittatas are one of the most loved egg dishes. It combines cheese, cream, meat, sautéed vegetables, and beaten eggs. Frittata is the Italian omelet but cooked a bit differently—beaten eggs mixed with a little liquid, cooked, and then filled with a vegetable, meat, and cheese.

The ingredients are similar to those of the omelet, but it is cooked in a skillet then finished in the oven.

Prep: 10 minutes

Cook: 30 minutes

Calories (240), fat (16.7), carbohydrates (5.5), protein: (16.7)

Ingredients

- 12 ounces ground breakfast sausage, turkey
- 2 bell peppers
- 12 eggs
- 1 cup lactose-free sour cream
- 1 teaspoon pink Himalayan salt

- 1 teaspoon black pepper
- 2 teaspoons butter
- 2 ounces shredded cheddar (optional)

Instructions

- Preheat the oven to 350°F.
- Blend eggs, the sour cream, salt, and pepper on high for 30 seconds.
- Heat a large skillet on medium heat, and once hot, add the butter.
- Slice the bell peppers into strips and throw them into the skillet to sauté until browned and tender for about 6 minutes.
- Remove the bell peppers from the skillet once browned.
- Put the turkey sausage in the skillet and stir while breaking up the meat until it is brown. This should take about eight minutes.
- Flatten the turkey on the bottom of the skillet and add the bell peppers over it evenly.
- Add the egg mix. Pour over everything.

- Place the skillet in the oven and bake for 30 minutes. If you want to add the cheese, sprinkle it over the frittata as soon as you take it out of the oven so it melts.

8. Ketogenic Breakfast Tacos

Prep: 15 minutes

Cook: 10 minutes

Total: 25 minutes

Sugar (2 g), fat (29 g), carbohydrates (4 g), protein (20 g)

Ingredients

- 3 ounces aged cheddar (Tillamook)
- 1 large pastured egg
- 2 slices sugar-free bacon, pastured
- 2 sprigs cilantro
- arugula, a handful
- 1 teaspoon ghee
- a pinch of salt, pepper, and turmeric

Instructions

- Cook bacon. Pan-fry it or pop it in the oven at 350°F until crispy.
- Shred the cheese with a cheese grater.
- Heat skillet on medium-high heat and then add the ghee into the skillet once it is hot.
- Sprinkle the cheese all around into the ghee in the skillet.
- The cheese will start melting almost instantly.
- Once the cheese has melted, crack the egg in the middle of the molten cheese and sprinkle salt, pepper, and turmeric on the yolk.
- Cook for 2 minutes until the egg begins to become opaque and the cheese begins to brown.
- Cook covered for 2 minutes. Seal with a tight-fitting lid and lower the heat.
- Remove. The egg should be fully cooked and the cheese crispy.

- Slide your cheese egg onto a chopping board or dish. Elevate the sides so that the shell cools and hardens and the sides stay up.
- Add the bacon, cilantro, and arugula.

9. *Crock-Pot Pumpkin Coconut Breakfast Bars*

Prep time: 20 minutes

Serves: 8

Ingredients

- 1 3/4 cup canned pumpkin puree
- 2/3 cup swerve sweetener
- 1 teaspoon raw apple cider vinegar
- 3 eggs, beaten
- 1 cup coconut flour
- 1 tablespoon pumpkin pie spice
- 1/2 tablespoon cinnamon

- 1/2 teaspoon baking soda

- 1/4 teaspoon salt

- 1/3 cup pecan, toasted and chopped

Instructions

1. Line the bottom of the Crock-Pot with parchment paper lightly oiled with cooking oil.

2. In a bowl, mix the pumpkin puree, sweetener, apple cider vinegar, and eggs.

3. In another bowl, mix the coconut flour, pumpkin pie spice, cinnamon, baking soda, and salt.

4. Pour the wet ingredients to the dry ingredients and fold until well mixed.

5. Pour the batter into the Crock-Pot and sprinkle with pecans.

6. Cover with lid. Cook for 3 hours on low or until a toothpick inserted in the middle comes out clean.

Nutrition Information

Calories per serving: 187.4

Carbohydrates: 8.5 g

Protein: 6 g

Fat: 17.2 g

Sugar: 2.5 g

Sodium: 165 mg

Fiber: 3 g

10. Overnight Eggs Benedict Casserole

Prep time: 25 minutes

Serves: 10

Ingredients

- 1 pound Canadian bacon, sliced

- 10 large eggs, beaten
- 1 cup milk
- salt and pepper to taste
- 6 egg yolks
- 2 tablespoons chives, chopped
- 1 1/2 sticks butter, cubed

Instructions

1. Spray cooking oil in the Crock-Pot's ceramic interior.
2. Take the bacon slices at the bottom of the Crock-Pot.
3. In a bowl, mix the eggs and milk. Season with salt and pepper to taste.
4. Pour over the bacon.
5. Close the lid and cook for 1 1/2 hours.

6. Open the lid and take the egg yolks on top. Sprinkle with chopped chives.

7. Continue cooking for another 1 1/2 hours or until the egg mixture is done.

8. While still warm, keep butter on top.

Nutrition Information

Calories per serving: 256

Carbohydrates: 2 g

Protein: 16.2 g

Fat: 21 g

Sugar: 0 g

Sodium: 734 mg

Fiber: 0.3 g

11. Crustless Crock-Pot Spinach Quiche

Prep time: 50 minutes

Serves: 6

Ingredients

- 1 tablespoon ghee
- 2 cups baby bella mushrooms, chopped
- 1 medium red bell peppers, sliced
- 1 package chopped spinach, drained
- 8 eggs, beaten
- 1 cup sour cream
- 1/2 teaspoon salt
- 1/4 teaspoon black pepper
- 1 1/2 cup cheddar cheese, shredded
- 2 tablespoons chives, chopped
- 1/2 cup almond flour
- 1/4 teaspoon baking soda

Instructions

1. Oil the slow cooker with cooking spray.

2. In a skillet, heat the ghee and sauté the mushrooms and bell peppers for 4 hours. Add the kale and cook for another minute. Set aside.

3. In a bowl, mix the eggs and sour cream. Season with salt and pepper. Stir in the cheese and chives. Add the almond flour and baking soda. Mix until well mixed. Stir in the vegetable mixture.

4. Pour the mixture in the Crock-Pot and cook on low for 5 hours or 3 hours on high.

Nutrition Information

Calories per serving: 383.1

Carbohydrates: 7.3 g

Protein: 15.1 g

Fat: 18 g

Sugar: 0 g

Sodium: 547 mg

Fiber: 3.2 g

12. *Cheesy and Eggy Breakfast Casserole*

Prep time: 35 minutes

Serves: 8

Ingredients

- 12 eggs, beaten
- 3/4 cup half-and-half
- 1/2 teaspoon red pepper flakes
- 1/2 teaspoon salt
- 1/4 teaspoon ground black pepper
- 1 cup cheddar cheese, shredded
- 1 cup Colby cheese, shredded
- 1/2 cup green onions, chopped

- 1 cauliflower head, cut into florets
- 1 pound pork sausages, cooked and sliced
- 1/2 cup red bell peppers, roasted and chopped

Instructions

1. Line the sides of the slow cooker with foil. Oil with cooking spray so that the mixture will not stick on the Crock-Pot.

2. In a mixing bowl, mix the eggs, half-and-half, red pepper flakes, salt, and black pepper. Add the cheeses, onions, and cauliflower florets.

3. Take the sausages at the bottom of the Crock-Pot.

4. Pour over the egg mixture and top with chopped roasted bell peppers.

5. Close the lid and cook for 3 hours or until a toothpick inserted in the middle comes out clean.

Nutrition Information

Calories per serving: 475

Carbohydrates: 5.2 g

Protein: 23 g

Fat: 26.7 g

Sugar: 0.2 g

Sodium: 791 mg

Fiber: 2.1 g

13. Broccoli and Tomatoes Casserole

Prep time: 30 minutes

Serves: 6

Ingredients

- 1 large broccoli, chopped

- 2 tablespoons butter
- Salt and pepper to taste
- 1 1/4 cups cooked bacon, crumbled
- 1 1/2 cups cherry tomatoes, halved
- 2 cups cheddar cheese, shredded
- 8 eggs, beaten
- 1/2 cup whole milk
- 1 bunch scallions, sliced

Instructions

1. Spray cooking spray on the interior of the Crock-Pot.
2. In a mixing bowl, toss the broccoli and butter. Season with salt and pepper to taste.
3. Press the vegetable mixture at the bottom of the Crock-Pot. Add the bacon and tomatoes on top. Add the cheddar cheese.

4. In a mixing bowl, mix the eggs and milk.

5. Pour the egg mixture over the vegetable layers. Sprinkle the scallions.

6. Close the lid and cook on low for 4 hours or until a toothpick inserted in the middle comes out clean.

Nutrition Information

Calories per serving: 486

Carbohydrates: 8.1

Protein: 21.3 g

Fat: 17 g

Sugar: 2.9 g

Sodium: 845 mg

Fiber: 5.4 g

14. *Simple Ham-and-Egg Casserole*

Prep time: 40 minutes

Serves: 6

Ingredients

- 4 tablespoons butter, melted
- 1/2 green bell pepper, diced
- 1/2 red bell pepper, diced
- 1 small onion, diced
- 1/2 cup ham, diced
- 1/2 cup cheese, shredded
- 6 eggs, beaten
- 1 tablespoon milk
- salt and pepper to taste

Instructions

1. Spray the Crock-Pot with cooking spray.
2. Take melted butter in the Crock-Pot.

3. Add the bell peppers, onions, ham, and cheese in layers.

4. In a mixing bowl, mix the eggs and milk. Season with salt and pepper.

5. Pour over the layers of vegetables and ham.

6. Close the lid and cook for 3 hours on low or until a toothpick inserted in the middle comes out clean.

Nutrition information

Calories per serving: 379.1

Carbohydrates: 7.2 g

Protein: 15 g

Fat: 20.4 g

Sugar: 1.4 g

Sodium: 744 mg

Fiber: 3.9 g

15. *Fluffy Breakfast Omelet*

Prep time: 25 minutes

Serves: 8

Ingredients

- 4 strips bacon, cooked and crumbled
- 1 small onion, chopped
- 2 bell peppers, chopped
- 1 small head broccoli, chopped
- 1/2 cup cheddar cheese, shredded
- 4 egg whites
- 8 eggs, beaten
- 3/4 cup milk
- 2 teaspoons mustard, ground
- 1/2 teaspoon garlic salt
- Salt and pepper to taste

Instructions

1. Oil the Crock-Pot with cooking spray.
2. Arrange in layers the bacon, onion, bell pepper, and broccoli.
3. Top with half of the cheddar cheese.
4. In a mixing bowl, beat the egg whites with a hand mixer until it forms stiff peaks. Set aside.
5. In another bowl, mix the eggs, milk, mustard, and garlic. Season with salt and pepper.
6. Fold the egg-white mixture into the milk mixture gently.
7. Pour over the vegetable mixture.
8. Top with the remaining cheese.
9. Close the lid and cook for 3 hours or until a toothpick inserted in the middle comes out clean.

Nutrition information

Calories per serving: 320

Carbohydrates: 6.5 g

Protein: 22.3 g

Fat: 23.2 g

Sugar: 1.9 g

Sodium: 700 mg

Fiber: 5.3 g

16. *Crock-Pot Mediterranean Frittata*

Prep time: 30 minutes

Serves: 8

Ingredients

- 8 eggs, beaten
- 1/3 cup milk
- 1 teaspoon dried oregano
- salt and pepper to taste

- 4 cups baby arugula rockets, rinsed and drained
- 1 1/4 cups red peppers, roasted and chopped
- 1/2 cup red onion, sliced thinly
- 3/4 cup goat cheese, crumbled

Instuctions

1. Spray cooking oil inside the Crock-Pot.
2. In a large bowl, mix the eggs, milk, and oregano. Season with salt and pepper.
3. Take the arugula leaves at the bottom of the Crock-Pot. Add the red peppers, onions and goat cheese.
4. Pour over the egg mixture.
5. Cook on low for 3 hours.
6. Serve warm.

Nutrition Information

Calories per serving: 416

Carbohydrates: 7.2 g

Protein: 18.3 g

Fat: 15.9 g

Sugar: 1.3 g

Sodium: 481 mg

Fiber: 4.8 g

17. *Spinach and Mozzarella Frittata*

Prep time: 15 minutes

Serves: 6

Ingredients

- 1 tablespoon extra-virgin olive oil
- 1/2 cup onion, diced
- 3 eggs, beaten

- 1 cup mozzarella cheese, divided

- 2 tablespoons milk

- Salt and pepper to taste

- 3 egg whites, beaten until stiff peaks form

- 1 cup baby spinach, rinsed

- 1 tomato, diced

Instructions

1. In a small skillet, heat oil and sauté the onions for 2 minutes. Set aside.

2. Spray the inside of the Crock-Pot with cooking spray.

3. In a bowl, mix the sautéed onions, eggs, mozzarella cheese, and milk. Season with salt and pepper to taste.

4. Fold the beaten egg whites to the egg mixture. Set aside.

5. Arrange the baby spinach and tomatoes at the bottom of the Crock-Pot.

6. Pour over the egg mixture.

7. Close the lid and cook for 3 hours on low or until a toothpick inserted in the middle comes out clean.

Nutrition Information

Calories per serving: 139

Carbohydrates: 4 g

Protein: 12 g

Fat: 8 g

Sugar: 2 g

Sodium: 435 mg

Fiber: 1 g

18. Artichoke Hearts and Roasted Pepper Frittata

Prep time: 30 minutes

Serves: 8

Ingredients

- 1 can artichoke hearts, drained and cut into small pieces
- 1 cup roasted red peppers, seeds removed and chopped
- 1/4 cup green onions, sliced
- 8 eggs, beaten
- 1/2 cup feta cheese, crumbled
- Salt and pepper to taste
- Chopped parsley for garnish

Instructions

1. Take the artichoke hearts into the oiled Crock-Pot.
2. Add the red peppers and green onions.

3. In a bowl, mix the eggs and cheese. Season with salt and pepper to taste.

4. Pour over the vegetables.

5. Sprinkle parsley on top.

6. Cook on low for 2 1/2 hours.

Nutrition Information

Calories per serving: 322

Carbohydrates: 8.1 g

Protein: 16 g

Fat: 14.2 g

Sugar: 0.6 g

Sodium: 486.2 mg

Fiber: 5.2 g

19. Sausage Cauliflower Breakfast Casserole

Prep time: 40 minutes

Serves: 10

Ingredients

- 1 head cauliflower, chopped finely
- 4 tablespoon unsalted butter, melted
- 2 teaspoons salt
- 1 pound breakfast sausage
- 6 green onions, chopped
- 12 large eggs, beaten
- 1/2 cup mozzarella cheese, shredded

Instructions

1. Take the chopped cauliflower at the bottom of the Crock-Pot. Pour butter and season with salt.
2. Take the sausages and onions on top of the cauliflower bed. Pour over the beaten eggs and top with mozzarella cheese.

3. Cook on low for 3 hours.

Nutrition Information

Calories per serving: 478

Carbohydrates: 5.7 g

Protein: 16.3 g

Fat: 22 g

Sugar: 0.5 g

Sodium: 550 mg

Fiber: 3.8 g

20. Greek Crock-Pot Breakfast Casserole

Prep time: 25 minutes

Serves: 12

Ingredients

- 12 eggs, beaten
- 1/2 cup milk
- 1/2 teaspoon salt

- 1/4 teaspoon black pepper
- 1 teaspoon onion powder
- 1 teaspoon garlic powder
- 1/2 cup sundried tomatoes, soaked overnight
- 1 cup baby bella mushrooms, sliced
- 2 cups spinach
- 1/2 cup feta cheese, shredded

Instructions

1. Lubricate the Crock-Pot with cooking spray.
2. Mix all ingredients in a bowl.
3. Pour the mixture in the Crock-Pot.
4. Cook on low for 4 hours.

Nutrition Information

Calories per serving: 397

Carbohydrates: 7.5 g

Protein: 16.3 g

Fat: 20.3 g

Sugar: 1.2 g

Sodium: 347 mg

Fiber: 3.7 g

21. Coconut Cranberry Quinoa Pudding

Prep time: 40 minutes

Serves: 10

Ingredients

- 3 cups coconut water
- 1 cup quinoa, uncooked
- 1 teaspoon vanilla extract
- 3 teaspoons stevia extract
- 1/3 cup coconut flakes

- 1/3 cup almonds, sliced
- 1/4 cup dried cranberries

Instructions

1. Take all ingredients inside the Crock-Pot.
2. Cook on low for 4 hours.
3. Serve warm.

Nutrition Information

Calories per serving: 246

Carbohydrates: 4 g

Protein: 8 g

Fat: 5 g

Sugar: 3 g

Sodium: 0 mg

Fiber: 5 g

22. *Crock-Pot Breakfast Lettuce Burritos*

Prep time: 30 minutes

Serves: 12

Ingredients

- 12 eggs, beaten
- 1 cup milk
- 1 cup diced ham
- salt and pepper to taste
- lettuce leaves
- cherry tomatoes, halved
- chives, chopped
- sour cream

Instructions

1. Spray the Crock-Pot with cooking spray.

2. In a bowl, mix all ingredients except the lettuce, cherry tomatoes, chives, and sour cream.

3. Cook on low for 4 hours.

4. After an hour, give the egg mixture a stir to create a scrambled-egg-like consistency.

5. Bring together the lettuce burritos by placing the egg mixture on top of the lettuce. Add tomatoes, chives, and sour cream.

Nutrition Information

Calories per serving: 275

Carbohydrates: 4.2 g

Protein: 12.3 g

Fat: 17.7 g

Sugar: 1.2 g

Sodium: 346 mg

Fiber: 2.3 g

23. Breakfast Three-Cheese Shrimps

Prep time: 15 minutes

Serves: 10

Ingredients

- 6 cups chicken stock
- 1 tablespoon garlic powder
- 1 tablespoon onion powder
- 1 teaspoon dried thyme
- salt and pepper to taste
- 1 cup cheddar cheese, shredded
- 4 ounces light cream cheese
- 1/2 cup Parmesan cheese, grated
- 1/2 teaspoon hot sauce
- 2 pounds raw shrimp

- chopped scallions for garnish

Instructions

1. Take all components except the scallions in the slow cooker.
2. Give a stir to incorporate everything.
3. Cook for 30 minutes or an hour on low.
4. Garnish with chopped scallions.

Nutrition Information

Calories per serving: 472

Carbohydrates: 1.2 g

Protein: 17.6 g

Fat: 32 g

Sugar: 0 g

Sodium: 870 mg

Fiber: 0.2 g

Lunch Recipes

1. Broccoli Chicken Zucchini Boats (2 servings)

Carbs (5 g), fat (34 g), protein (30 g)

This is a perfect lunch when you need something a little out of the ordinary. The fillings are perfect and come out with all the flavors.

Ingredients

- 10 ounces zucchini
- 2 tablespoons of butter
- 3 ounces shredded cheddar cheese
- 1 cup broccoli
- 6 ounces shredded rotisserie chicken
- 2 tablespoons sour cream
- 1 stalk green onion
- salt and pepper

Method of Preparation

- Preheat the oven to 400°F and cut the zucchini into halves, lengthwise.

- Using a spoon, scoop out most of the zucchini until you are left with a shell that is about a centimeter thick

- Pour a tablespoon of melted butter into each zucchini boat and season with salt or pepper and place in the oven. This gives the zucchini time to cook as you prepare the filling. This takes about twenty minutes.

- Shred your chicken using two forks so as to pull the meat apart. Measure out 6 ounces and place the rest in the refrigerator for another meal.

- Cut up your broccoli florets until they are bite-sized.

- Mix the chicken and broccoli with sour cream to keep them moist and creamy. Season.

- As soon as the zucchini has cooked, take them out and add the chicken and broccoli filling.

- Sprinkle cheddar cheese on top of your chicken and broccoli and pop them back into the oven for another 15 minutes until the cheese is melted and browning.

- Garnish with chopped green onion.

2. Cheese-Stuffed Bacon-Wrapped Hot Dogs (6 hot dogs)

Carbs (0.3 g), fat (34.5 g), protein (16.8 g), calories (380)

This takes about 10 minutes to prepare.

Ingredients

- 6 hot dogs

- 12 slices of bacon

- 2 ounces cheddar cheese

- 1/2 teaspoon garlic powder

- 1/2 teaspoon onion powder
- salt and pepper

Instructions

- Heat the oven to 400°F. Slit all the hot dogs to create space for cheese.
- Slice 2 ounces cheddar cheese into small and long rectangles. Stuff them into the hotdogs.
- Tightly wrap one slice of bacon around the hotdog
- Go on and tightly wrap the second slice of bacon around the hot dog. Make sure it slightly overlaps with the first slice.
- Poke each side of the bacon and hot dog with a toothpick so as to secure the bacon in place.
- You then set on a wire rack that's on top of a cookie sheet. Season with garlic powder, onion powder, salt, and pepper.

- Bake for between 35 and 40 minutes or until the bacon becomes crispy. You can also broil the bacon on top if needed.

- Serve with some nice creamed spinach.

3. Bacon, Avocado, and Chicken Sandwich (2 servings)

Carbs (2 g), fat (28.3 g), protein (22 g), calories (361)

Ingredients

Keto cloud bread:

- 3 large eggs
- 3 ounces cream cheese
- 1/8 teaspoon cream of tartar
- 1/4 teaspoon salt
- 1/2 teaspoon garlic powder

Filling:

- 1 tablespoon mayonnaise

- 1 teaspoon sriracha
- 2 bacon slices
- 3 ounces chicken
- 2 pepper jack cheese slices
- 2 grape tomatoes
- 1/4 medium avocado

Method of Preparation

- Preheat the oven to 300°F. Start by separating 3 eggs into 2 clean dry bowls.
- Mix the cream of tartar and salt with the egg whites.
- Use an electric mixer to whip the whites until they become soft and foamy.
- In a separate bowl, mix 3 ounces of cubed cream cheese with the egg yolks and beat until they become pale yellow.
- Fold the egg whites into the yolks.

- On a parchment-paper-lined baking sheet, spoon 1/4 cup of the keto cloud bread batter.

- Use a spatula to gently press the tops of the keto cloud bread to form squares. You then sprinkle the tops with garlic powder and bake for about 25 minutes.

- As the keto cloud bread is baking, cook the chicken and bacon with salt and pepper.

- You arrange the sandwich by combining mayo and sriracha and spreading it on the underside of one keto cloud bread. Add the chicken into the mayo mixture.

- Add the two slices of pepper jack cheese and the bacon. Nestle some halved grape tomatoes and spread the mashed avocado on top. Season to taste and top with the other keto cloud bread.

4. Crispy Tofu and Bok Choy Salad (3 servings)

Carbs (5.7 g), fat (35 g), protein (25 g), calories (442)

Tofu that is baked is quite delicious. You get a rich cube that is full of flavor and crunchy on the outsides. Furthermore, raw bok choy is fantastic. It is crunchy and offers a distinct taste to the salad.

Ingredients

Oven baked tofu:

- 15 ounces extra firm tofu
- 1 tablespoon soy sauce
- 1 tablespoon sesame oil
- 1 tablespoon water
- 2 teaspoons minced garlic
- 1 tablespoon rice wine vinegar
- juice made from half a lemon

Bok choy salad:

- 9 ounces bok choy
- 1 stalk of green onion
- 2 tablespoons chopped cilantro
- 3 tablespoons coconut oil
- 2 tablespoons soy sauce
- 1 tablespoon sambal olek
- 1 tablespoon peanut butter
- juice from half a lime
- 7 drops liquid stevia

Instructions

- Begin by pressing the tofu. Place the tofu in a kitchen towel and put something heavy over it. It takes about 4–6 hours to dry out. However, you may need to change the kitchen towel when halfway done.

- After pressing the tofu, work on the marinade. Mix all the ingredients for the marinade. That is soy sauce, sesame oil, water, garlic, vinegar, and lemon.

- Chop the tofu into squares and place them in a plastic bag together with the marinade. Let it marinate for at least half an hour. However, overnight is preferred.

- Preheat the oven to 350°F. Place the tofu on a baking sheet lined with parchment paper. Bake for half an hour.

- When the tofu is cooked, start on the bok choy salad. Chop the cilantro and spring onion.

- You then mix all the other ingredients together apart from lime juice and bok choy. You then add cilantro and the spring onion. You can also microwave the coconut oil for about ten seconds so that it melts.

- When the tofu is almost cooked, add the lime juice into the salad dressing and mix together.

- Chop the bok choy into small pieces.

Remove the tofu from the oven and assemble the salad with tofu, bok choy, and sauce.

5. Avocado Tuna Melt Bites (12 pieces)

Carbs (0.8 g), fat (11.8 g), protein (6.2 g), calories (135)

Their crispy outside combines with the soft creamy filling on the inside.

Ingredients

- 10 ounces canned and drained tuna
- 1/4 cup mayonnaise
- 1 medium avocado, cubed
- 1/4 cup Parmesan cheese
- 1/3 cup almond flour

- 1/2 teaspoon garlic powder
- 1/4 teaspoon onion powder
- salt and pepper
- 1/2 cup coconut oil for frying

Instructions

- Drain a can of tuna and add to a large-sized container where everything will be mixed.
- Add mayonnaise, Parmesan cheese, and spices to the tuna. Mix well.
- Slice the avocado into half and cube it.
- Add avocado into the tuna mixture and fold together. Try not to mash the avocado into the mixture.
- Form the tuna mixture into balls and roll into almond flour, covering them completely. Set aside.

- Heat the coconut oil in a pan over medium heat. As soon as it's hot, add the tuna balls and fry until all sides are crisp.

- Remove from the pan and serve.

6. Portobello Bun Cheeseburgers

Mushrooms, technically, are fungi. However, just like vegetables, portobello mushrooms are packed with essential nutrients and are a great addition to the keto diet.

Unprocessed foods, like mushrooms, help reduce the risk of many health conditions, including obesity, diabetes, and heart disease.

Portobello mushrooms contain two types of dietary fiber (beta-glucans and chitin), which play an important role in weight management. With these dietary fibers, satiety increases and appetite decreases.

Health Benefits of Mushrooms

- Promotes heart health
- Great source of B vitamins

- Boosts immunity
- Low in calories
- Contains disease-fighting antioxidants
- Helps combat inflammation
- Great source of fiber

Prep: 5 minutes

Cook: 15 minutes

Total time: 20 minutes

Calories (336), fat (22.8 g), carbohydrates (5.8 g), carbs (4 g), protein (29.1 g)

Ingredients

- 1 pound grass-fed 80/20 ground beef
- 1 tablespoon Worcestershire sauce
- 1 teaspoon pink Himalayan salt
- 1 teaspoon black pepper
- 1 tablespoon avocado oil
- 6 portobello mushroom caps (destemmed, rinsed, and dabbed dry)
- 6 slices sharp cheddar cheese

Instructions

- Mix ground beef, salt, pepper, and Worcestershire sauce.
- Make the mixture into burger patties.
- Heat avocado oil over medium heat in a large pan and then add portobello mushroom caps.
- Cook for about 3–4 minutes on each side then remove.
- Cook the burger patties in the same pan, 4 minutes on one side and 5 minutes on the other until you get the desired doneness.
- Add cheese to the patties and then cover with a lid to melt the cheese. Do this for about 1 minute.

Garnish Options

- Romaine
- Sugar-free barbecue sauce
- Sliced dill pickles
- Spicy brown mustard

7. Crock-Pot Beef Roast

Prep time: 20 minutes

Serves: 6

Ingredients

- 2 pounds beef chuck roast, trimmed of excess fat
- 1 1/2 teaspoons salt
- 3/4 teaspoon black pepper
- 2 tablespoons fresh basil, chopped
- 1 large yellow onion, chopped
- 4 cloves garlic, minced
- 2 bay leaves
- 2 cups beef stock

Instructions

1. Pat dry the beef roast with a paper towel and rub with salt, pepper, and chopped basil.

2. Take inside the Crock-Pot and spread the onion, garlic, and bay leaves.

3. Pour over the beef stock.

4. Close the lid and cook on low for 10 hours until tender.

Nutrition Information

Calories per serving: 234

Carbohydrates: 2.4 g

Protein: 33.1 g

Fat: 10.3 g

Sugar: 0.9 g

Sodium: 758.2 mg

Fiber: 0.5 g

8. Chipotle Barbecue Chicken

Prep time: 20 minutes

Serves: 5

Ingredients

- 1/4 cup water
- 1 1/4 ounce boneless chicken breasts, skin removed
- 1 1/4 ounce boneless chicken thighs, skin removed
- salt and pepper to taste
- 2 tablespoons chipotle Tabasco sauce
- 1 onion, chopped
- 4 tablespoons unsalted butter
- 1 cup tomato sauce
- 1/3 cup apple cider vinegar
- 1/2 cup water
- 2 tablespoons yellow mustard
- 1/4 teaspoon garlic powder

Instructions

1. Take all ingredients in a Crock-Pot.

2. Give everything a stir so that the chicken is coated with the sauce.

3. Close the lid and cook on low for 8 hours.

Nutrition Information

Calories per serving: 482

Carbohydrates: 3 g

Protein: 29.4 g

Fat: 18.7 g

Sugar: 0 g

Sodium: 462 mg

Fiber: 0.3 g

9. Spicy Shredded Chicken Lettuce Wraps

Prep time: 15 minutes

Serves: 8

Ingredients

- 4 chicken breast, skin and bones removed
- 1 cup tomato salsa
- 1 teaspoon onion powder
- 1 can green chilies, diced
- 1 tablespoon Tabasco sauce
- 2 tablespoons lime juice, freshly squeezed
- salt and pepper to taste
- 2 large heads iceberg lettuce, rinsed

Instructions

1. Take the chicken breast in the Crock-Pot.
2. Pour over the tomato salsa, onion powder, green chilies, Tabasco sauce, and lime juice. Season with salt and pepper to taste.

3. Close the lid and cook for 10 hours.

4. Shred the chicken meat using a fork.

5. Take on top of lettuce leaves.

6. Garnish with sour cream, tomatoes, or avocado slices if needed.

Nutrition Information

Calories per serving: 231

Carbohydrates: 3 g

Protein: 23 g

Fat: 12 g

Sugar: 0.5 g

Sodium: 375 mg

Fiber: 2 g

10. Bacon Cheeseburger Casserole

Prep time: 50 minutes

Serves: 8

Ingredients

- 2 pounds ground beef
- 1/2 onion, sliced thinly
- 1/2 teaspoon salt
- 1/2 teaspoon black pepper
- 1 (15-ounce) can cream of mushroom soup
- 1 (15-ounce) can cheddar cheese soup
- 1/2 pounds bacon, cooked and crumbled
- 2 cups cheddar cheese, grated

Instructions

1. Brown the ground beef and onions in a skillet over medium heat. Season with salt and pepper to taste.

2. Take the beef in the Crock-Pot and add the cream of mushroom soup and cheese soup.

3. Pour in the bacon and half of the cheddar cheese. Give a stir.

4. Cook on low for 4 hours.

5. An hour before the cooking time is over. Add the remaining cheese on top.

Nutrition Information

Calories per serving: 322

Carbohydrates: 2 g

Protein: 36 g

Fat: 21 g

Sugar: 0 g

Sodium: 271 mg

Fiber: 1.3 g

11. Crock-Pot Ranch Chicken

Prep time: 55 minutes

Serves: 6

Ingredients

- 2 pounds boneless chicken breasts
- 3 tablespoons dry ranch dressing mix
- 3 tablespoons butter
- 4 ounces cream cheese

Instructions

1. Take the chicken in the Crock-Pot. Pour the ranch dressing and rub on the chicken.
2. Add the butter and cream cheese.
3. Close the lid and cook for 7 hours on low.
4. Shred the chicken before serving.

Nutrition Information

Calories per serving: 266

Carbohydrates: 0 g

Protein: 33 g

Fat: 12.9 g

Sugar: 0 g

Sodium: 167 mg

Fiber: 0 g

12. Coconut Cilantro Shrimp Curry

Prep time: 40 minutes

Serves: 4

Ingredients

- 1 can light coconut milk
- 15 ounces water
- 1/2 cup Thai red curry sauce
- 2 1/2 teaspoons lemon juice

- 1 teaspoon garlic powder
- 1/4 cup cilantro
- salt and pepper to taste
- 1 pound shrimps, heads removed only

Instructions

1. Take the coconut milk, water, and curry sauce in the Crock-Pot.
2. Stir in the lemon juice, garlic powder, and cilantro. Season with salt and pepper to taste.
3. Cook on high for 23 hours.
4. Add the shrimps and cook on high for 10 minutes.

Nutrition Information

Calories per serving: 211

Carbohydrates: 2 g

Protein: 18.2 g

Fat: 22 g

Sugar: 0 g

Sodium: 135 mg

Fiber: 0.8 g

13. *Crock-Pot Butter Masala Chicken*

Prep time: 45 minutes

Serves: 8

Ingredients

- 1 tablespoon olive oil
- 9 cloves of garlic, crushed
- 2 teaspoons *garam masala*
- 2 pounds boneless chicken breasts, cut into strips
- 1 can light coconut milk
- 1 can tomato paste

- 1/2 teaspoon cayenne pepper
- 1 teaspoon dried coriander
- 1 tablespoon paprika
- 1 teaspoon turmeric powder
- 1 teaspoon cumin powder
- 1 1/2 teaspoons salt

Instructions

1. Heat olive oil in a skillet over medium flame and sauté the garlic for 1 minute. Add the garam masala and cook for another minute or until fragrant. Set aside.
2. Take the chicken in the Crock-Pot and add the garlic and garam masala mixture. Stir to coat the chicken meat.
3. Add the rest of the ingredients and cook on low for 7 hours.

Nutrition Information

Calories per serving: 520

Carbohydrates: 2.3 g

Protein: 32.7 g

Fat: 28 g

Sugar: 0 g

Sodium: 342 mg

Fiber: 0.8 g

14. *Kashmiri Lamb Curry*

Prep time: 40 minutes

Serves: 6

Ingredients

- 4 dried red chili peppers
- 3 long green fresh chili peppers
- 1 teaspoon cumin seeds

- 1 teaspoon garam masala
- 1 piece ginger root, peeled and grated
- 5 cloves garlic, crushed
- 1/4 cup unsweetened coconut meat, shredded
- 3 tomatoes, chopped
- 6 tablespoons vegetable oil
- 2 large onions, sliced
- 2 pounds lamb meat
- 1/2 teaspoon ground turmeric
- 1 cup plain yogurt
- 1/4 cup cilantro, chopped
- 1 cup water
- salt and pepper to taste

Instructions

1. Take the chilies, cumin seeds, garam masala, ginger, garlic, coconut, and tomatoes in a blender and pulse until smooth. Set aside.

2. In a skillet, heat vegetable oil and sauté the onions and lamb meat for 3 minutes.

3. Transfer the meat mixture in the Crock-Pot. Pour in chili paste mixture on top of the lamb.

4. Add the turmeric, yogurt, cilantro, and water. Season with salt and pepper.

5. Cook on low for 7 hours until tender.

Nutrition Information

Calories per serving: 489

Carbohydrates: 3 g

Protein: 25 g

Fat: 40 g

Sugar: 0 g

Sodium: 166 mg

Fiber: 2.5 g

15. Chicken with Bacon Gravy

Prep time: 35 minutes

Serves: 4

Ingredients

- 1 1/2 pounds chicken breasts, bones and skin removed
- 1/4 teaspoon pepper
- 1 teaspoon salt
- 1 teaspoon minced garlic
- 1 teaspoon dried thyme
- 6 slices of bacon, cooked and crumbled
- 1 1/2 cups water

- 2/3 cup heavy cream

Instructions

1. Take all ingredients except the heavy cream in the Crock-Pot.
2. Close the lid and cook on low for 6 hours.
3. Add the heavy cream and continue cooking for another hour.

Nutrition Information

Calories per serving: 359

Carbohydrates: 0.9 g

Protein: 21 g

Fat: 25 g

Sugar: 0 g

Sodium: 0 mg

Fiber: 0 g

16. *Garlic Butter Chicken with Cream Cheese*

Prep time: 20 minutes

Serves: 8

Ingredients

- 2 1/2 pounds chicken breast
- 1 stick butter, softened
- 8 cloves garlic, sliced in half
- 1 onion, sliced
- 1 1/2 teaspoon salt
- 8 ounces cream cheese
- 1 cup chicken stock

Instructions

1. Take the chicken in the Crock-Pot and add the butter.
2. Stir in the garlic and onions. Season with salt.
3. Cook on low for 6 hours.

4. Meanwhile, prepare the cream cheese sauce by mixing together cream cheese and chicken stock in a saucepan. Heat over medium flame and stir until the sauce has reduced.

5. Pour over the chicken.

Nutrition Information

Calories per serving: 463

Carbohydrates: 2 g

Protein: 22.4 g

Fat: 35 g

Sugar: 0 g

Sodium: 674 mg

Fiber: 0.6 g

17. Cheesy Adobo Chicken

Prep time: 30 minutes

Serves: 6

Ingredients

- 1 pound chicken breasts, bones removed but with skin on
- 1 tablespoon butter
- 1/2 cup tomatoes, sliced
- 2 tablespoons adobo sauce
- 1/2 cup milk
- 3/4 cup cheddar cheese, shredded

Instructions

1. Take all ingredients in the Crock-Pot.
2. Give a stir and cook on low for 8 hours.
3. Use a fork to shred the chicken.

Nutrition Information

Calories per serving: 493

Carbohydrates: 0 g

Protein: 25.8 g

Fat: 33.9 g

Sugar: 0 g

Sodium: 375 mg

Fiber: 0 g

18. Ketogenic Chicken Tikka Masala

Prep time: 25 minutes

Serves: 6

Ingredients

- 1 1/2 pounds chicken thighs, bone in and skin on
- 2 tablespoons olive oil
- 2 teaspoons onion powder
- 5 teaspoons garam masala
- 3 cloves of garlic
- 3 tablespoons tomato paste

- 1 inch gingerroot, grated
- 2 teaspoons smoked paprika
- 1 cup tomatoes, diced
- 1 cup coconut milk
- 1 cup heavy cream
- salt to taste
- fresh cilantro for garnish

Instructions

1. Take all ingredients except the cilantro in the Crock-Pot.
2. Mix everything until the spices are incorporated well.
3. Close the lid and cook on low for 8 hours.
4. Garnish with cilantro once cooked.

Nutrition Information

Calories per serving: 493

Carbohydrates: 4.3 g

Protein: 26.6 g

Fat: 41.2 g

Sugar: 1 g

Sodium: 457 mg

Fiber: 2 g

19. Balsamic Chicken Thighs

Prep time: 30 minutes

Serves: 8

Ingredients

- 1 teaspoon dried basil
- 2 teaspoons minced onion
- 1 teaspoon garlic powder
- 1/2 teaspoon salt

- 1/2 teaspoon black pepper
- 8 boneless chicken breasts
- 1 tablespoon extra-virgin olive oil
- 4 cloves garlic, minced
- 1/2 cup balsamic vinegar
- parsley for garnish

Instructions

1. In a small bowl, mix the dried basil, onion, garlic, salt, and pepper.
2. Rub the spice mixture onto the chicken. Set aside.
3. Take olive oil in the Crock-Pot and sprinkle minced garlic.
4. Arrange the chicken piece on top of the oil and garlic.
5. Pour balsamic vinegar.
6. Cook on low for 8 hours.

7. Garnish with parsley once cooked.

Nutrition Information

Calories per serving: 133

Carbohydrates: 5.6 g

Protein: 20.1 g

Fat: 4 g

Sugar: 3 g

Sodium: 832 mg

Fiber: 0.1 g

20. Chicken Lo Mein

Prep time: 40 minutes

Serves: 6

Ingredients

- 1 1/2 pounds chicken, sliced into strip
- 1 tablespoon coconut aminos

- 1/2 teaspoon sesame oil
- 1/2 teaspoon garlic paste
- 2 cloves garlic, minced
- 1 teaspoon ginger, minced
- 1 bunch bok choy, washed and sliced
- 12 ounces kelp noodles
- salt and pepper to taste
- 3/4 cup chicken broth
- 1 tablespoon rice vinegar
- 1 teaspoon red pepper chili flakes

Instructions

1. In a small bowl, mix the chicken, coconut aminos, sesame oil, and garlic paste. Let it marinate for 30 minutes inside the fridge.

2. Cook the marinated chicken in the Crock-Pot on high for 2 hours. Set aside.

3. Take the garlic, ginger, and bok choy at the bottom of the Crock-Pot. Add the chicken and kelp noodles on top. Season with salt and pepper to taste.

4. In a bowl, mix the chicken broth, rice vinegar, and red pepper flakes.

5. Pour over the chicken mixture and cook for 30 minutes on high.

Nutrition Information

Calories per serving: 174

Carbohydrates: 3.1 g

Protein: 24.5 g

Fat: 8.1 g

Sugar: 0.5 g

Sodium: 436 mg

Fiber: 1.6 g

21. Ethiopian Doro Watt Chicken

Prep time: 35 minutes

Serves: 6

Ingredients

- 1 teaspoon chili powder
- 1 teaspoon sweet paprika
- 1 tablespoon salt
- 1 teaspoon ground coriander
- 1/2 teaspoon ground ginger
- 1/8 teaspoon ground cardamom
- 1/8 teaspoon fenugreek powder
- 1/8 teaspoon nutmeg
- 1/8 teaspoon allspice
- 1 whole chicken, sliced into different parts

- 1/2 cup butter

- 2 large onions, chopped

- 1 clove of garlic, minced

- 8 hard-boiled eggs, shells removed

- 1/2 cup water

Instructions

1. Mix the first 9 ingredients in a bowl. Use this spice mix and rub it on the chicken parts. Let the chicken marinate for 30 minutes in the fridge.

2. Take the butter in the Crock-Pot and add the onion and garlic. Take the chicken pieces. Arrange the hard-boiled eggs randomly on top of the chicken.

3. Pour water.

4. Close the lid and cook on low for 8 hours.

Nutrition Information

Calories per serving: 315

Carbohydrates: 4 g

Protein: 19 g

Fat: 25 g

Sugar: 0 g

Sodium: 698 mg

Fiber: 0.8 g

Snack and Side Recipes

1. Crock-Pot Keto Chocolate Cake

Prep time: 20 minutes

Serves: 12

Ingredients

- 3/4 cup stevia sweetener
- 1 1/2 cups almond flour
- 1/4 cup protein powder, chocolate or vanilla flavor

- 2/3 cup cocoa powder, unsweetened
- 1/4 teaspoon baking powder
- 1/4 teaspoon salt
- 1/2 cup unsalted butter, melted
- 4 large eggs
- 3/4 cup heavy cream
- 1 teaspoon vanilla extract

Instructions

1. Grease the ceramic insert of the Crock-Pot.

2. In a bowl, mix the sweetener, almond flour, protein powder, cocoa powder, baking powder, and salt.

3. Add the butter, eggs, cream, and vanilla extract.

4. Pour the batter in the Crock-Pot and cook on low for 3 hours.

5. Allow it to cool before slicing.

Nutrition Information

Calories per serving: 253

Carbohydrates: 5.1 g

Protein: 17.3 g

Fat: 29.5 g

Sugar: 1.2 g

Sodium: 361 mg

Fiber: 2.4 g

2. *Keto Crock-Pot Chocolate Lava Cake*

Prep time: 30 minutes

Serves: 12

Ingredients

- 1 1/2 cups stevia sweetener, divided
- 1/2 cup almond flour
- 5 tablespoons unsweetened cocoa powder
- 1/2 teaspoon salt
- 1 teaspoon baking powder

- 3 whole eggs
- 3 egg yolks
- 1/2 cup butter, melted
- 1 teaspoon vanilla extract
- 2 cups hot water
- 4 ounces sugar-free chocolate chips

Instructions

1. Grease the inside of the Crock-Pot.
2. In a bowl, mix the stevia sweetener, almond flour, cocoa powder, salt, and baking powder.
3. In another bowl, mix the eggs, egg yolks, butter, and vanilla extract. Pour in the hot water.
4. Pour the wet ingredients to the dry ingredients and fold to create a batter.
5. Add the chocolate chips last.

6. Pour into the greased Crock-Pot and cook on low for 3 hours.

7. Allow to cool before serving.

Nutrition Information

Calories per serving: 157

Carbohydrates: 5.5 g

Protein: 10.6 g

Fat: 13 g

Sugar: 0.2 g

Sodium: 155 mg

Fiber: 2.6 g

3. Lemon Crock-Pot Cake

Prep time: 15 minutes

Serves: 8

Ingredients

- 1/2 cup coconut flour

- 1 1/2 cups almond flour
- 3 tablespoons stevia sweetener
- 2 teaspoons baking powder
- 1/2 teaspoon xanthan gum
- 1/2 cup whipping cream
- 1/2 cup butter, melted
- 1 tablespoon juice, freshly squeezed
- zest from one large lemon
- 2 eggs

Instructions

1. Grease the inside of the Crock-Pot with butter or cooking spray.
2. Mix together coconut flour, almond flour, stevia, baking powder, and xanthan gum in a bowl.
3. In another bowl, combine the whipping cream, butter, lemon juice,

lemon zest, and eggs. Mix until well combined.

4. Pour the wet ingredients to the dry ingredients gradually and fold to create a smooth batter.

5. Spread the batter in the Crock-Pot and cook on low for 3 hours or until a toothpick inserted in the middle comes out clean.

Nutrition Information

Calories per serving: 350

Carbohydrates: 11.1 g

Protein: 17.6 g

Fat: 32.6 g

Sugar: 0.9 g

Sodium: 224 mg

Fiber: 4.9 g

4. Keto Basic Vanilla Cake in a Crock-Pot

Prep time: 25 minutes

Serves: 12

Ingredients

- 1 1/2 cups almond flour
- 3/4 cup stevia sweetener
- 2/3 cup protein powder, vanilla powder
- 1/4 teaspoon salt
- 2 teaspoons baking powder
- 1/2 cup unsalted butter, melted
- 3/4 cup heavy cream
- 4 large eggs
- 1 teaspoon vanilla extract

Instructions

1. Grease the insert of the Crock-Pot with cooking spray.

2. In a bowl, mix the almond flour, sweetener, protein powder, salt, and baking powder.

3. In another bowl, combine the butter, heavy cream, eggs, and vanilla extract.

4. Pour the wet ingredients to the dry ingredients and fold to create a smooth batter.

5. Pour into the greased Crock-Pot.

6. Cook on low for 3 hours.

7. Let it cool before serving.

Nutrition Information

Calories per serving: 162

Carbohydrates: 4.1 g

Protein: 11.6 g

Fat: 12.3 g

Sugar: 2.3 g

Sodium: 154 mg

Fiber: 0.5 g

5. *Mocha Pudding Cake*

Prep time: 60 minutes

Serves: 6

Ingredients

- 3/4 cup butter, cut into chunks
- 2 ounces unsweetened chocolate, chopped
- 1/2 cup heavy cream
- 2 tablespoons instant coffee
- 1 teaspoon vanilla extract
- 1/3 cup almond flour
- 4 tablespoons cocoa powder, unsweetened
- 1/8 teaspoon salt

- 5 large eggs

- 2/3 cup stevia sweetener

Instructions

1. Grease the Crock-Pot pot with cooking spray or butter.

2. In a double boiler, melt the butter and unsweetened chocolate over medium heat. Once melted, remove from heat and allow to cool.

3. In a small bowl, combine the heavy cream, coffee, and vanilla extract.

4. In another bowl, combine the almond flour, cocoa powder, and salt.

5. Beat the eggs in a large bowl and add the stevia sweetener until slightly thickened or until it turns pale yellow.

6. To the egg mixture, pour in the melted chocolate. Whisk until

combined. Add the flour mixture gradually while continuously whisking.

7. Pour in the coffee mixture last. Whisk until combined.

8. Pour the batter into the Crock-Pot.

9. Place a paper towel on top of the Crock-Pot before closing the lid.

10. Cook on low for 3 hours.

Nutrition Information

Calories per serving: 414

Carbohydrates: 3.8 g

Protein: 10.9 g

Fat: 38.9 g

Sugar: 13 g

Sodium: 542 mg

Fiber: 0.9 g

6. Cinnamon Blondie Pecan Bars

Prep time: 55 minutes

Serves: 16

Ingredients

- 1 cup stevia sweetener
- 6 tablespoons unsalted butter, melted
- 3 large eggs
- 2 teaspoons vanilla extract
- 1 1/2 cups almond flour
- 1/4 teaspoon salt
- 1 tablespoon cinnamon
- 1 teaspoon baking powder
- 2 tablespoons unsalted butter
- 1/4 cup heavy whipping cream
- 1 cup pecans, chopped

Instructions

1. Grease the Crock-Pot with butter.

2. In a bowl, combine the stevia sweetener and melted butter. Add in the eggs and vanilla extract.

3. Use a hand mixer to combine the ingredients.

4. In another bowl, combine the almond flour, salt, baking powder, and cinnamon.

5. Mix the wet ingredients to the dry ingredients until combined.

6. Pour the dough in the Crock-Pot and press to form a dense bar.

7. Cook on low for 3 hours.

8. Meanwhile, mix the butter, whipping cream and pecans in a saucepan. Allow to boil and reduce slightly.

9. Once the bars are cooked, pour over the pecan sauce.

Nutrition Information

Calories per serving: 190.6

Carbohydrates: 1.9 g

Protein: 4.42 g

Fat: 20.56 g

Sugar: 0.5 g

Sodium: 163 mg

Fiber: 0 g

7. Crock-Pot Dark Chocolate Cake

Prep time: 40 minutes

Serves: 10

Ingredients

- 1 cup almond flour

- 1/2 cup cocoa powder

- 1/2 cup stevia sweetener

- 3 tablespoons whey protein powder, unflavored

- 1 1/2 teaspoons baking powder

- 1/4 teaspoon salt

- 3 large eggs

- 2/3 cup unsweetened almond milk

- 6 tablespoons butter, melted

- 3/4 teaspoon vanilla extract

- 1/3 cup sugar-free chocolate chips

Instructions

1. Grease the Crock-Pot with butter.

2. In a medium bowl, whisk the almond flour, cocoa powder, stevia powder, and whey protein. Add in the baking powder and salt.

3. In another bowl, combine the eggs, almond milk, butter, and vanilla extract.

4. Pour the wet ingredients to the dry ingredients and whisk until the batter is smooth.

5. Add the chocolate chips last.

6. Pour the batter in the Crock-Pot and bake on low for 3 hours.

Nutrition Information

Calories per serving: 205

Carbohydrates: 8.42 g

Protein: 7.37 g

Fat: 16.79 g

Sugar: 0.3 g

Sodium: 230 mg

Fiber: 4.1 g

8. Easy Crock-Pot Cheesecake

Prep time: 35 minutes

Serves: 6

Ingredients

- 3 (8-ounce) cream cheese, room temperature
- 1 cup stevia sweetener
- 3 eggs
- 1/2 tablespoon vanilla extract

Instructions

1. Grease the Crock-Pot with butter.
2. In a mixing bowl, mix the cream cheese and stevia sweetener.
3. Use a hand mixer to mix everything.
4. Add the eggs and vanilla extract.
5. Pour the mixture into the Crock-Pot and cook on low for 3 hours.

Nutrition Information

Calories per serving: 264

Carbohydrates: 3 g

Protein: 9.1 g

Fat: 15.8 g

Sugar: 2.6 g

Sodium: 157 mg

Fiber: 0 g

Dessert Recipes

1. Pumpkin Pecan Pie Ice Cream (4 one-cup servings)

Or for extra decadence, one can add 3–4 ounces cream cheese to this recipe.

Ingredients

- 1/2 cup cottage cheese
- 1/2 cup pumpkin puree

- 1 teaspoon pumpkin spice
- 2 cups coconut milk
- 1/2 teaspoon xantham gum
- 3 large egg yolks
- 1/3 cup erythritol
- 20 drops liquid stevia
- 1 teaspoon maple extract
- ½ cup pecans, toasted and chopped
- 2 tablespoons salted butter

Instructions

- Chop the toasted pecans and put on the stove with butter. Leave it over low heat until the butter turns brown. In case you don't have toasted pecans, place in a pan and toast over low heat for between 7 and 10 minutes.

- Place all the ingredients into a container that can accommodate the immersion blender.

- Use your immersion blender to blend all the ingredients together into a mixture that is smooth.

- Add the mixture to your ice-cream machine.

- Once your butter turns brown and the pecans have soaked up some of the butter, place inside the ice-cream machine.

- Follow the churning instructions as per your ice-cream manufacturer's instructions.

> **Nutrient intake per serving:**
>
> Carbs: 4.3 g
>
> Fat: 22.3 g
>
> Protein: 6.5 g
>
> Calories: 248

2. Ketogenic Amaretti Cookies (16 cookies)

These are delicate and sweet. Each one is soft and full of almond and fruity flavors. This recipe uses strawberry jam.

Ingredients

- 1 cup almond flour
- 2 tablespoons coconut flour
- ½ teaspoon baking powder

- 1/4 teaspoon baking powder
- 1/4 teaspoon cinnamon
- Half a teaspoon of salt
- 1/2 cup erythritol
- 2 large eggs
- 4 tablespoons coconut oil
- 1/2 teaspoon vanilla extract
- 1/2 teaspoon almond extract
- 2 tablespoons sugar-free jam
- 1 tablespoon organic shredded coconut

Instructions

- Preheat the oven to 350°F. Mix all the dry ingredients and whisk.
- Add in the wet ingredients and mix well. Use a whisk or hand mixer.
- Form the cookies on a parchment-paper-lined baking sheet. Add an

indent at the middle of each cookie using your finger or the back of a measuring spoon.

- Bake for about 15 minutes or until the cookies turn golden or crack slightly.

- Let the cookies cool on a wire rack and fill each indent with sugar-free jam.

- Lastly, sprinkle some shredded coconut on top of each cookie.

- Dish out and serve.

Nutrient intake per serving:

Carbs: 1.2 g

Fat: 7.9 g

Protein: 2.4 g

Calories: 86

These bars are easy to make and can be frozen or refrigerated depending on what you need.

3. No-Bake Coconut Cashew Bars (8 servings)

Ingredients

- 1 cup almond flour
- 1/4 cup melted butter
- 1/4 cup sugar-free maple syrup
- 1 teaspoon cinnamon
- a pinch of salt
- 1/2 cup cashews
- 1/4 cup shredded coconut

Instructions

- Mix the melted butter and almond flour in a large bowl.
- Add cinnamon, salt, and sugar-free maple syrup and mix properly.

- You then add the shredded coconut and mix again.

- Roughly chop 1/2 cup of cashews, whether raw or roasted. Add to the coconut cashew bar dough. Mix well.

- Line a baking dish with parchment paper and spread the coconut cashew bar dough in an even layer. You can add some more shredded coconut and cinnamon on top.

- Place them in the refrigerator and chill for at least two hours. However, overnight is recommended. As soon as they are chilled, slice them into bars. Serve and enjoy!

Nutrient intake per serving:

Carbs: 4 g

Fat: 17.6 g

Protein: 4 g

Calories: 189

4. Ketogenic Chocolate-Covered Macaroons (12 macaroons)

These macaroons are sweet with a nice coconut, almond, and chocolate flavor.

Ingredients

- 1 cup unsweetened shredded coconut
- 1 large white egg
- 1/4 cup erythritol

- 1/2 teaspoon almond extract

- a pinch of salt

- 20 grams sugar-free chocolate

- 2 tablespoons coconut oil

Instructions

- Preheat the oven to 350°F and spread a cup of shredded and unsweetened coconut into a thin layer on a parchment-paper-lined baking sheet. As soon as the oven is hot enough, place the coconut in to toast up a little for about five minutes.

- As the coconut toasts, beat the egg white until it's foamy.

- Add the erythritol and a pinch of salt as you continue to mix.

- You then add the almond extract for a twist on normal coconut macaroons.

- Once the coconut flakes have toasted and cooled, add them in and fold everything together.

- Use an ice-cream scoop or your hands to tightly pack little balls of macaroon batter and gently place them on a parchment-paper-lined baking sheet. Bake until they are golden. This should take around 15 minutes.

- As they bake, make the chocolate drizzle by melting coconut oil and the sugar-free chocolate. Continuously stir to make sure the chocolate doesn't burn.

- When the macaroons are out of the oven, drizzle your chocolate over each one of them.

> **Nutrient intake per serving:**
>
> Carbs: 1 g
>
> Fat: 7.3 g
>
> Protein: 1 g
>
> Calories: 73

5. Ketogenic Chocolate Peanut Butter Tarts (4 servings)

Ingredients

Crust:

- 1/4 cup flaxseeds
- 2 tablespoons almond flour
- 1 tablespoon erythritol

- 1 large egg white

Top layer:

- 1 medium avocado
- 4 tablespoons cocoa powder
- 1/4 cup erythritol
- 1/2 teaspoon vanilla extract
- 1/2 teaspoon cinnamon
- 2 tablespoons heavy cream

Middle layer:

- 4 tablespoons peanut butter
- 2 tablespoons butter

Instructions

- Preheat the oven to 350°F. Make your crust by grinding up 1/4 cup flaxseeds until they are finely ground.

- Add the rest of the crust ingredients to the ground flaxseeds. Blend until well mixed.

- Press the crust mixture into the tart pans and up the sides. Bake for about 8 minutes until set.

- As the crust bakes, prepare the top layer by mixing all the ingredients in a blender and blend until smooth and creamy.

- After removing the crusts from the oven, let them cool as you prepare your peanut butter layer. Melt the peanut butter and butter in the microwave or a small pan over the stove until well mixed and soft.

- Pour the melted layer of peanut butter onto the tart crusts and place in the fridge for half an hour until set.

- As soon as the top of the peanut butter layer is set, add the chocolate avocado layer on top. Smooth it out and refrigerate for an hour.

Nutrient intake per serving:

Carbs: 3.9 g

Fat: 26.8 g

Protein: 9.8 g

Calories: 305

6. Peaches and Cream Dessert

Peaches and cream dessert is a delicious summer delicacy and fit perfectly in the keto diet with the right calories count.

Prep time: 10 minutes

Ingredients

- 4 tablespoons unsalted butter, softened
- 6 ounces softened cream cheese
- 1 cup frozen peaches, warmed lightly
- 3/4 scoop peaches and cream ketone supplement
- 3 1/2 tablespoon fruit sweetener, separated

Instructions

- In a medium-sized bowl with a hand mixer, mix butter, cream cheese, peaches, peaches and cream ketone supplement, and 3 tablespoons of monk fruit sweetener until well-combined.
- Scoop mixture into a silicone mold. Top each fat bomb with remaining monk fruit sweetener.
- Place mold in the freezer and freeze for 4 hours.
- Once frozen, remove fat bombs from silicone mold and enjoy!
- Freeze time: 4 hours.

Nutrition

Calories: 43

Fat: 4.2

Carbohydrates: 1

Net carbs: 0.9

Protein: 0.5

> **Nutrient intake per cookie:**
> - Fat: 43 g
> - Carbs: 4.21 g
> - Net carbs: 0.9 g
> - Protein: 0.5 g

7. Lemon Cashew Cookies

Lemon cashew cookies are low in carbohydrates and are a nutritious dessert for the keto diet, but because cashews are high in carbs, use only raw cashew butter with no added sugar. In place of cashew nuts, you can also use macadamia nuts, which are high in fat (80% monounsaturated) and are rich in antioxidants, minerals, and vitamins.

Prep time: 10 minutes

Cook time: 12 minutes

Total time: 22 minutes

Yield: 12

Category: snacks

Cuisine: American

Ingredients
- 1 cup cashew butter

- 2 eggs
- zest of 1 lemon
- juice of 1 lemon
- 1/2 teaspoon vanilla extract
- 6–10 drops liquid stevia (or 1/4 teaspoon powdered stevia)
- 1/4 teaspoon baking soda

Instructions

- Preheat oven to 350°F.
- Wash the lemon and dry it thoroughly. Use a fine grater to zest the lemon rind into a large bowl. Be sure to get the entire colorful outer layer of the lemon. Then cut open the lemon and squeeze the juice into the bowl being careful not to let any seeds in the bowl.
- Add the cashew butter, eggs, vanilla, baking soda, and stevia to the bowl and mix with a fork or spoon until all of the ingredients are fully blended.
- The consistency will be like a thick, viscous batter, which is a bit thicker than nut butter but a bit thinner than the usual cookie dough. Take 12 small heaps of the

batter and place onto a cookie sheet, shaping into a cookie shape.
- Bake at 350°F for about 10–15 minutes. Let cool before serving.

Nutrient intake per cookie:

Calories: 140 g

Sugar: 3 g

Fat: 9 g

Carbohydrates: 4 g

Protein: 4 g

Tips about the Desserts and Ingredients

Benefits of peaches:
- Peaches have 17% daily recommended value in vitamin C per serving, which boosts immunity.
- Peaches are low in saturated fat and cholesterol.
- They are a good source of vitamin E, vitamin K, niacin, and copper.

- They have vitamin A, which offers B-carotenes that convert to retinol, which is essential for sharp eyesight
- They are abundant in potassium to aid in the digestion of food, heart-rate regulation, and the lowering of blood pressure.
- Iron in peaches is required for red blood cell formation.
- Magnesium helps to prevent stress and anxiety and keeps the nervous system calm.
- The combination of phosphorous and calcium strengthens bones and teeth.
- Phenolic compounds containing anti-inflammatory and anti-obesity properties help fight metabolic syndromes.

Dinner Recipes

1. Low-Carb Walnut-Crusted Salmon (2 servings)

In the ketogenic diet, fatty fish has been proven to lower levels of cholesterol and aid with the overall health. This recipe is easy to prepare and super tasty. It takes under 15 minutes to prepare.

Ingredients

- 1/2 cup of walnuts
- 2 tablespoons sugar-free maple syrup
- 1/2 tablespoon Dijon mustard
- 1/4 teaspoon dill
- 2 (3-ounce) salmon fillets
- 1 tablespoon olive oil
- salt and pepper

Instructions

- Preheat the oven to 350°F. Add half a cup of walnuts to the food processor.
- Add two tablespoons of maple syrup and the spices.
- Add a tablespoon of mustard.
- Pulse this in the food processor until it is paste-like.
- Heat a pan or skillet with a tablespoon of oil until very hot. Thoroughly dry the salmon fillets and place them skin-down in the pan. Let it sear for about 3 minutes, undisturbed.

- As it sears, add the walnut mixture to the top side of the salmon fillets.
- After that, transfer them to an oven and bake for about 8 minutes.
- Serve with fresh spinach and enjoy. You can sprinkle a little bit of smoked paprika.

Nutrient intake per serving:
Carbs: 3 g
Fat: 43 g
Protein: 20 g
Calories: 373

2. Keto Hot-Chili Soup (4 servings)
Ingredients

- 1 teaspoon coriander seeds
- 2 tablespoons olive oil
- 2 sliced chili peppers
- 2 cups chicken broth

- 2 cups water
- 1 teaspoon turmeric
- 1/2 teaspoon ground cumin
- 4 tablespoons tomato paste
- 16 ounces chicken thighs
- 2 tablespoons butter
- 1 medium avocado
- 2 ounces queso fresco
- 4 tablespoons fresh chopped cilantro
- juice from half a lime
- salt and pepper

Instructions

- Cut and set the chicken thighs to cook in an oiled pan. Season it with salt and pepper. You then leave it aside to rest.
- In 2 tablespoons of olive oil, heat up the coriander seeds to release more flavor.
- Once they are fragrant, add in the sliced chili peppers to add their flavor to the oil.
- You then add in the broth and water. Let it simmer and season. Add turmeric, ground cumin, and salt and pepper to taste.

- As the soup simmers, add in the tomato paste and butter. Stir so that it melts and mixes. Let the soup simmer for between 5 and 10 minutes.
- Lower the heat on the stove and the juice from half the lime.
- Place 4 ounces of chicken thighs into the bottom of the bowl so that you are able to pour soup over it.
- Ladle the soup for serving. Garnish with a quarter of an avocado into each bowl, 1/2 ounce of queso fresco, and cilantro.

Nutrient intake per serving:

Carbs: 5.8 g

Fat: 27.8 g

Protein: 28 g

Calories: 396

3. Slow-Cooker Ketogenic Chicken Tikka Masala (5 servings)

Ingredients

- 1 (1/2-pound) chicken thighs, bone in, skin on
- 1 pound chicken thighs, boneless, skinless
- 2 tablespoons olive oil
- 2 teaspoons onion powder
- 3 cloves minced garlic
- 1 inch grated gingerroot
- 3 tablespoons tomato paste
- 5 teaspoons garam masala
- 2 teaspoons smoked paprika
- 4 teaspoons of kosher salt
- 10 ounces diced tomatoes, canned
- 1 cup heavy cream
- 1 cup coconut milk
- fresh chopped cilantro
- 1 teaspoon guar gum

Instructions

- Debone the chicken on the bone-in chicken thighs. Chop all the chicken pieces into bite-sized pieces. Ensure that you keep the skin for the pieces that have it.

- Add the chicken to a slow cooker and grate an inch of ginger over the top.
- Add all the dry spices into the slow cooker and mix properly.
- Add canned diced tomatoes and tomato paste into the slow cooker and mix well once more.
- Finally, add 1/2 cup of coconut milk and mix well. Cook over low heat for 6 hours or 3 hours over high heat.
- Once the slow cooker is over, add the remainder of the coconut milk, heavy cream, and guar gum and mix well into the chicken. This will help the curry thicken nicely.
- Serve over cauliflower rice or a veggie of your choice.

Nutrient intake per serving:

Carbs: 5.8 g

Fat: 41.2 g

Protein: 26 g

Calories: 493

4. Barbecue Bacon Cheeseburger Waffles (2 servings)

This meal is dense with calories.

Ingredients

Waffles:

- 5 ounces cheddar cheese
- 2 large eggs
- 1 cup cauliflower crumbles
- 1/4 teaspoon garlic powder
- 1/4 teaspoon onion powder
- 4 tablespoons almond flour
- 3 tablespoons Parmesan cheese
- salt and pepper

The topping:

- 4 ounces ground beef

- 4 slices of chopped bacon
- 4 tablespoons sugar-free barbecue sauce
- 1 1/2 ounces cheddar cheese
- salt and pepper

Instructions

- Shred 3 ounces of cheese. You will use half for the waffle and half on top.
- Measure out the cauliflower crumbles over a scale or use a cup.
- Mix in half of the cheddar cheese, Parmesan cheese, eggs, almond flour, and spices.
- Slice the bacon thinly over medium to high heat.
- As soon as the bacon is partially cooked, add in the beef.
- Add any excess grease from the pan into the waffle mixture that you set aside.
- Use an immersion blender to blend the waffle mixture into a paste that is thick.
- Add half of the mixture to the waffle iron and cook until crisp. Repeat for the second waffle.

- As the waffles cook, add in the sugar-free barbecue sauce to the bacon and ground mixture of the beef.
- Assemble the waffles together by adding half of the ground beef mixture and half of the remaining cheddar cheese to the top of the waffle
- Broil for about two minutes until the cheese is nicely melted over the top.
- Serve immediately. You may slice up green onion to sprinkle over the top.

5. *Bacon Cheeseburger Casserole (6 servings)*

Ingredients

- 1 pound ground beef
- 3 slices of bacon
- 1/2 cup of almond flour
- 256 grams cauliflower, riced
- 1 tablespoon psyllium husk powder
- 1/2 teaspoon garlic powder
- 1/2 teaspoon onion powder
- 2 tablespoons reduced sugar ketchup
- 1 tablespoon Dijon mustard
- 2 tablespoons mayonnaise

- 3 large eggs
- 4 ounces cheddar cheese
- salt and pepper

Instructions

- Preheat the oven to 350°F. Put rice cauliflower in the food processor and add dry ingredients. Mix well.
- Put bacon and ground beef in the food processor until crumbly. Cook over medium to high heat. Season with salt and pepper.
- Shred the cheese as the meat cooks. Once the meat is done, mix all the ingredients in a large bowl and add half of the cheddar cheese.
- Add eggs, mayo, ketchup, and mustard to the mixture. Use a fork or hands to mix everything well.
- Press the mixture into a 9×9 baking pan lined with parchment paper. You then top with the other half of the cheddar cheese.
- Place on the top rack and bake for 25–30 minutes. For additional crisp on top,

broil for around 3 minutes or until browned.
- Remove from oven and let it cool for between five and ten minutes.
- Slice and serve with additional toppings.

6. Shrimp Stir-Fry

Shrimp stir-fry is a great low-carb, high-fat keto meal that you can have ready within half an hour—shrimp healthily sautéed in bacon. Serve with a keto-friendly vegetable like cauliflower rice as a side dish to beef up nutrients. The portion of fat used is keto healthy and the bacon boosts the fat content, which ensures sufficient fat stores for fuel.

Ingredients
- 16 ounces (or 1 pound) shrimps, peeled with tail on
- 2 inches gingerroot
- 4 stalks scallion or green onion
- 2 garlic cloves
- 4 baby bella mushrooms
- 1 inch lemon rind
- 2 teaspoon sea salt (or to taste)

- 3 tablespoons bacon fat
- 12 ounces frozen cauliflower rice
- 2 tablespoons MCT oil
- coconut aminos
- sesame seeds
- chili flakes

Instructions

- Preheat oven to 400°F.
- Drizzle MCT oil liberally on cauliflower on a sheet pan and sprinkle the salt.
- Place in the oven once it reaches 400°F and cook for 10 minutes.
- Cut scallion into pieces of about 1 inch. Peel enough lemon rind. Slice garlic and ginger.
- Sauté the onions, ginger, and garlic in bacon fat on medium heat in a large skillet until they are aromatic and soft.
- Once they are soft, add the shrimp and sauté. Keep stirring until the shrimps turn pink and are coiled.
- Add coconut aminos and more salt (if you want). Keep stirring for 3 minutes and then turn off the heat.

- Serve the sautéed shrimp over the cauliflower rice and garnish with chili flakes, green onion, and sesame seeds.

Nutrient intake per serving:

Calories: 357

Fat: 24.8

Carbs: 9

Protein: 24.7

7. Bone Broth

Broth soup is nutrient-rich. It boosts immunity and reduces inflammation. Simmer animal bone in water infused with herbs and vinegar to melt out the collagen in the bone and marrow.

Prep time: 1 hour

Cook: 23 hours

Ingredients

- 4 pounds animal bone pastured (or 3 pounds pastured whole chicken)
- 10 cups filtered water (or as you deem enough)

- 2 tablespoons peppercorns
- 1 lemon
- 3 tablespoons turmeric
- 1 teaspoon salt
- 2 tablespoons apple cider vinegar
- 3 bay leaves (or as you want)

Instructions

- Preheat oven to 400°F.
- Roast bones or chicken for 45 minutes on a sheet pan and sprinkle salt.
- Transfer to a slow cooker or an electric pressure cooker.
- Add apple cider vinegar, bay leaves, peppercorns, and water.
- Simmer on low for 24–48 hours. If pressure cooking, do high for 2 hours then turn to slow cook for 12 hours.
- After that, sieve the broth over a large bowl.
- Discard everything else other than the strained broth.
- Divide the broth into three bowls or jars each with 2 cups.

- Add a teaspoon of turmeric and a slice or 2 of lemon to each of the 3 containers.
- Refrigerate and eat within 5 days.
- Warm on low heat.

Nutrient intake per cup serving:
Calories: 70
Sugar: 0
Fat: 4
Carbs: 1
Protein: 6

8. Baked Cauliflower with Bacon and Cheese

This is a satiating meal high in fat and low on carbs combining cauliflower nutrient with cheese and bacon.

Prep time: 15 minutes
Cook time: 45 minutes
Total time: 1 hour
Yield: 4

Ingredients

- 1 large head cauliflower, cut into florets
- 2 tablespoon butter
- 1 cup heavy cream
- 2 ounces cream cheese
- 1 1/4 cups shredded sharp cheddar cheese, separated
- salt and pepper to taste
- six slices bacon, cooked and crumbled
- 1/4 cup chopped green onions

Instructions

- Preheat oven to 350°F.
- In a large pot of boiling water, blanch cauliflower florets for 2 minutes. Drain cauliflower.
- In a medium pot, melt together butter, heavy cream, cream cheese, 1 cup of shredded cheddar cheese, salt, and pepper until well-combined.
- In a baking dish, add cauliflower florets, cheese sauce, all but 1 tablespoon crumbled bacon, and all but 1 tablespoon green onions. Stir together.

- Top with remaining shredded cheddar cheese, crumbled bacon, and green onions.
- Bake until cheese is bubbly and golden and cauliflower is soft, about 30 minutes.
- Serve immediately and enjoy!

Nutrient intake per serving:
Calories: 498
Fat: 45
Carbs: 5.8
Net carbs: 4.1
Protein: 13.9

9. Miracle Noodle Stuffed with Chicken

Miracle noodle stuffed with chicken is an effortless easy dinner fix—a dish combining different foods in one. Miracle noodles, also known as Shirataki noodles, are zero-carb Japanese noodles. Depending on the type of miracle noodle, they are very low carb to no carb. They are made of 3% glucomannan fiber, which slows down glucose absorption (thus blood sugar regulating), and 97% water.

Cook time: 25–35 minutes

Total time: 45 minutes

Ingredients

- 1 pack miracle noodle angel hair pasta
- 1 tablespoon avocado oil
- 2 cups spinach
- 2 ounces mozzarella cheese
- 1 pound boneless skinless chicken breast
- 1 teaspoon salt
- 1 teaspoon pepper
- 1 teaspoon white pepper

Instructions

- Preheat oven to 400°F.
- While oven is heating up, prepare the miracle noodles by draining them and adding them to a pot of boiling water. Let it simmer in water for 10 minutes.
- While the miracle noodles are simmering, sautée spinach and avocado oil in a pan on medium heat.

- Place chicken on cutting board and cut slices in them hasselback-style, enough room to stuff with pasta and spinach.
- Drain the miracle noodles and add to the spinach pan. Mix in cheese. Mix all together.
- Add spoonfuls of miracle noodles, spinach, and cheese to the pockets cut in the chicken breasts.
- Once all the pockets are stuffed, place the chicken on a baking sheet covered with parchment paper.
- Place in the oven to bake for 25–35 minutes or until fully cooked.

Nutrient intake per serving:

1 chicken breast (6 ounces)

Calories: 363

Fat: 13 g

Carbohydrates:

Net carbs: 2.3 g

Fiber: 1.7 g

Protein: 60 g

10. Easy White Turkey Chili

Preparation: 5 minutes

Cook time: 15 minutes

Total time: 20 minutes

Ingredients

- 1 pound organic ground turkey (or ground beef, lamb, or pork)
- 2 cups riced cauliflower
- 2 tablespoon coconut oil
- 1/2 a Vidalia onion
- 2 garlic cloves
- 2 cups full-fat coconut milk (or heavy cream)
- 1 tablespoon mustard
- 1 teaspoon salt, black pepper, thyme, celery salt, garlic powder

Instructions

- In a large pot, heat the coconut oil.
- In the meantime, mince the onion and garlic. Add it to the hot oil.
- Stir for 2–3 minutes then add in the ground turkey.
- Break up with the spatula and stir constantly until crumbled.

- Add in the seasoning mix and riced cauliflower and stir well.
- Once the meat is browned add in the coconut milk, bring to a simmer and reduce for 5–8 minutes, stirring often.
- At this point, it's ready to serve, or you can let it reduce by half until thick and serve as a dip.
- Mix in shredded cheese for an extra thick sauce.

Topping suggestions:
- Avocado
- Jalapenos
- Bacon
- Shredded aged cheddar cheese
- Cherry tomatoes
- Hot sauce

11. Bacon Cheddar Broccoli Salad

Prep time: 35 minutes

Serves: 6

Ingredients
- 6 slices raw bacon, chopped

- 1 bunch steamed broccoli, cut into small florets
- 3/4 cup mayonnaise
- 2 tablespoons apple cider vinegar
- 3 packets stevia powder
- 1/2 cup cheddar cheese
- 1/4 cup onion, chopped
- 1/4 cup sunflower seeds, roasted

Instructions

1. Take a parchment paper on the bottom of the Crock-Pot. Take the bacon in the Crock-Pot.
2. Cook on low for 8 hours or until the bacon is crispy.
3. Take the bacon in a bowl and add the steamed broccoli.
4. In another bowl, add the mayonnaise, apple cider vinegar, and stevia powder. Mix well.
5. Pour over the bacon and broccoli and toss to mix.
6. Add the cheddar cheese, onion, and sunflower seeds.

Nutrition Information

Calories per serving: 231

Carbohydrates: 8.1 g

Protein: 16 g

Fat: 15.3 g

Sugar: 2.4 g

Sodium: 751 mg

Fiber: 3 g

12. Chicken Yellow Curry

Prep time: 40 minutes

Serves: 6

Ingredients

- 1 1/2 pounds chicken breasts, skin and bones removed
- 6 cups mixed vegetables (preferably broccoli and cauliflower)
- 1 can full-fat coconut milk
- 1 cup crushed tomatoes
- 1 tablespoon cumin
- 2 teaspoons ground coriander
- 2 teaspoons ground ginger
- 2 teaspoons ground ginger powder
- 1 teaspoon cinnamon
- 1/2 teaspoon cayenne pepper

- 1 cup water
- salt to taste

Instructions

1. Take the chicken and vegetables in the Crock-Pot.
2. Add the rest of the ingredients and stir to mix everything.
3. Close the lid and cook on low for 6 hours.

Nutrition Information

Calories per serving: 425

Carbohydrates: 3 g

Protein: 23 g

Fat: 31.4 g

Sugar: 0 g

Sodium: 371.4 mg

Fiber: 0.9 g

13. Thai Whole Chicken Soup

Prep time: 25 minutes

Serves: 10

Ingredients

- 1 whole chicken
- 1 stalk lemongrass, cut into chunks

- 20 fresh basil leaves
- 5 thick slices of ginger
- 1 tablespoon salt (or more if needed)
- 1 lime, sliced

Instructions

1. Take the whole chicken inside the Crock-Pot.
2. Surround it with lemongrass stalks, 10 basil leaves, and ginger.
3. Fill the Crock-Pot with water until the maximum line. Season with salt.
4. Cook on low for 10 hours or until the chicken is tender.
5. Serve with lime and the remaining basil leaves.

Nutrition Information

Calories per serving: 475

Carbohydrates: 2 g

Protein: 42 g

Fat: 12 g

Sugar: 0 g

Sodium: 278 mg

Fiber: 0.5 g

14. Lemongrass and Coconut Chicken Drumsticks

Prep time: 15 minutes

Serves: 6

Ingredients

- 10 drumsticks, skin removed
- salt and pepper to taste
- 1 stalk lemongrass, cut into 5-inch-long sticks
- 3 tablespoon extra-virgin olive oil
- 1 thumb-sized ginger
- 4 cloves garlic, minced
- 2 tablespoons fish sauce
- 1 cup coconut milk
- 3 tablespoons coconut aminos
- 1 teaspoon five-spice powder
- 1 large onion, sliced thinly
- 1/4 cup fresh scallions, chopped

Instructions

1. Take the chicken drumstick in a bowl and season with salt and pepper. Set aside.
2. In a blender, take the lemongrass, oil ginger, garlic, fish sauce, coconut

milk, aminos, and five-spice powder. Blend until a smooth paste is formed.
3. Pour the paste or sauce into the marinated chicken and mix well. Allow it to marinate for another 2 hours.
4. Take the onion in the Crock-Pot and add the marinated chicken.
5. Cook on low for 8 hours.
6. Sprinkle with scallions on top.

Nutrition Information

Calories per serving: 528

Carbohydrates: 2 g

Protein: 32 g

Fat: 27 g

Sugar: 0 g

Sodium: 325 mg

Fiber: 0.8 g

15. Crock-Pot Beef Stroganoff

Prep time: 30 minutes

Serves: 8

Ingredients

- 2 pounds beef stew meat

- 2 teaspoons salt
- 1/2 teaspoon black pepper
- 1 teaspoon garlic powder
- 3 tablespoons extra-virgin olive oil
- 2 teaspoons paprika
- 1 teaspoon thyme
- 1 teaspoon onion powder
- 8 ounces mushrooms, sliced
- 1 small onion, sliced
- 1/3 cup coconut cream
- 2 teaspoons vinegar

Instructions

1. Season the beef stew meat with salt and pepper. Add the garlic powder, oil, paprika, thyme, and onion powder. Stir to mix all ingredients. Let the beef marinate for 2 hours inside the fridge.
2. Take the mushrooms and onion in the Crock-Pot and take the seasoned beef on top.
3. Close the lid and cook on low for 8 hours.

4. Once the meat is nearly done, add the coconut cream and vinegar. Adjust the seasoning if needed.

Nutrition Information

Calories per serving: 381

Carbohydrates: 2 g

Protein: 27.9 g

Fat: 24.5 g

Sugar: 0 g

Sodium: 0 mg

Fiber: 0.9 g

16. Spaghetti Squash with Shrimp Scampi

Prep time: 30 minutes

Serves: 4

Ingredients

- 2 cups chicken broth
- 1 small onion, chopped
- 2 1/2 teaspoon lemon-garlic seasoning
- 1 tablespoon butter or ghee
- 3 pounds spaghetti squash, cut crosswise and seeds removed

- 3/4 pounds shrimp, shelled and deveined
- salt and pepper to taste

Instructions

1. Pour broth in the Crock-Pot and stir in the lemon-garlic seasoning, onion, and butter.
2. Take the spaghetti squash and cook on high for hours.
3. Once cooked, remove the spaghetti squash from the Crock-Pot and run a fork through the meat to create the strands.
4. Take the squash strands back to the Crock-Pot and add the shrimps.
5. Season with salt and pepper.
6. Continue cooking on high for 30 minutes or until the shrimps have turned pink.

Nutrition Information

Calories per serving: 363.3

Carbohydrates: 1 g

Protein: 33 g

Fat: 21.2 g

Sugar: 0 g

Sodium: 276.2 mg

Fiber: 0.1 g

17. *Crock-Pot Garlic and Shrimps*

Prep time: 20 minutes

Serves: 10

Ingredients

- 3/4 cup extra-virgin olive oil
- 6 cloves of garlic, sliced
- 1 teaspoon smoked Spanish paprika
- 1 teaspoon salt
- 1/4 teaspoon black pepper
- 1/4 teaspoon red pepper flakes, crushed
- 2 pounds raw shrimp, shells removed and deveined
- 1 tablespoon parsley, minced

Instructions

1. In a small bowl, mix together olive oil, garlic, paprika, salt, pepper, and red pepper flakes.
2. Take the shrimp in the Crock-Pot and pour the spice mixture.

3. Stir to mix all ingredients.
4. Cook on low for 1 hour.
5. Garnish with parsley.

Nutrition Information

Calories per serving: 429

Carbohydrates: 1 g

Protein: 18 g

Fat: 24.5 g

Sugar: 0 g

Sodium: 211 mg

Fiber: 0 g

18. Pork Stew with Oyster Mushrooms

Prep time: 25 minutes

Serves: 4

Ingredients

- 2 tablespoon coconut oil
- 1 medium onion, chopped
- 1 clove of garlic, chopped
- 2 pounds pork loin, cut into cubes
- salt and pepper to taste
- 2 tablespoons oregano
- 2 tablespoons dried mustard
- 1/2 teaspoon ground nutmeg

- 1 1/2 cups bone broth
- 2 pounds oyster mushroom, rinsed
- 1/4 cup full-fat coconut milk
- 1/4 cup ghee
- 3 tablespoon capers

Instructions

1. In a skillet, melt the coconut oil over medium flame. Sauté the onion and garlic until fragrant. Add the pork loin and brown all sides. Season with salt and pepper to taste.
2. Transfer the sautéed meat, garlic, and onions in the Crock-Pot.
3. Add the oregano, mustard, nutmeg, bone broth, and oyster mushrooms.
4. Give a stir and cook on low for 10 hours.
5. Before the meat is nearly cooked, add the coconut milk and ghee.
6. Once done cooking, garnish with capers.

Nutrition Information

Calories per serving: 734
Carbohydrates: 12.5 g

Protein: 50.4 g

Fat: 48.9 g

Sugar: 2.3 g

Sodium: 1118 mg

Fiber: 7.9 g

19. Easy Crock-Pot Pork Loin

Prep time: 40 minutes

Serves: 12

Ingredients

- 5 pounds pork loin
- salt and pepper to taste
- 2 onions, chopped
- 3 cups beef broth

Instructions

1. Season the pork loin with salt and pepper.
2. Take inside the Crock-Pot and arrange the onions around the roast.
3. Pour the beef broth.
4. Cook on low for 10 hours until tender.

Nutrition Information

Calories per serving: 372

Carbohydrates: 0 g

Protein: 37.5 g

Fat: 23.4 g

Sugar: 0 g

Sodium: 261 mg

Fiber: 0 g

20. *Sticky Chicken Wings*

Prep time: 20 minutes

Serves: 6

Ingredients

- 3 tablespoons coconut aminos
- 2 tablespoons garlic, minced
- 1 tablespoon ginger, minced
- 1 teaspoon sesame oil
- 1/4 teaspoon salt
- 1 tablespoon xanthan gum
- 3 pounds chicken wings
- 2 tablespoons Chinese five-spice powder
- 3/4 teaspoon red pepper flakes
- Toasted sesame seeds for garnish

Instructions

1. Mix all ingredients except the sesame seeds.
2. Stir to coat the chicken wings.
3. Cook on low for 6 hours.
4. Garnish with sesame seeds.

Nutrition Information

Calories per serving: 475

Carbohydrates: 3 g

Protein: 31.8 g

Fat: 21 g

Sugar: 0 g

Sodium: 274 mg

Fiber: 0.9 g

21. Chicken and Kale Tortilla Stew

Prep time: 55 minutes

Serves: 6

Ingredients

- 4 cups of kale, stems removed and chopped
- 6 cups chicken broth
- 2 large chicken breasts
- 1 can crushed tomatoes
- 1 can sweetcorn

- 1/4 cup lime juice, freshly squeezed
- 1 can green chilies
- 2 tablespoons minced garlic
- 1 teaspoon cumin powder
- 2 tablespoons chili powder
- 1 teaspoon paprika
- 2 teaspoons garlic powder
- 1/4 cup Greek yogurt

Instructions

1. Take all ingredients except the Greek yogurt in the Crock-Pot.
2. Give a stir to mix all ingredients.
3. Cook on low for 5 hours.
4. Add the Greek yogurt and continue cooking on high for another hour.

Nutrition Information

Calories per serving: 362

Carbohydrates: 10 g

Protein: 25 g

Fat: 10 g

Sugar: 1.5 g

Sodium: 159 mg

Fiber: 6.3 g

22. Italian Chicken with Zucchini Noodles

Prep time: 1 hour and 10 minutes

Serves: 6

Ingredients

- 1/2 cup chicken broth
- 1 teaspoon Italian seasoning
- 4 teaspoons tomato paste
- 1 pound chicken breast
- 2 tomatoes, chopped
- 1 1/2 cups asparagus
- 1 cup snap peas, halved
- salt and pepper to taste
- 4 zucchini noodles, cut into noodle-like strips
- 1 cup commercial pesto
- Parmesan cheese for garnish
- Basil for garnish

Instructions

1. Take the chicken broth, Italian seasoning, tomato paste, chicken breasts, tomatoes, asparagus, and peas in the Crock-Pot. Give a swirl

and season with salt and pepper to taste.
2. Close the lid and cook on low for 6 hours. Let it cool before assembling.
3. Assemble the noodles by placing the chicken mixture on top of the zucchini noodles. Add commercial pesto and garnish with Parmesan cheese and basil leaves.

Nutrition Information

Calories per serving: 429.7

Carbohydrates: 6 g

Protein: 32 g

Fat: 26 g

Sugar: 0.4 g

Sodium: 0 mg

Fiber: 4.2 g

Chapter 6
Keto Meal Prep on a Budget

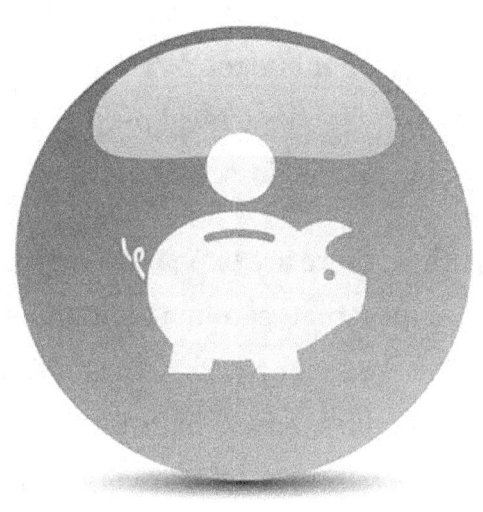

Chapter 6: Keto Meal Prep on a Budget

As much as there is a perception out there that the ketogenic diet is expensive, it isn't really true. It is possible to be on a keto diet comfortably on a budget. We shall learn in this chapter how to do keto meal prep on a budget of $50 weekly or even less.

The truth is, there are expensive ingredients for some recipes that can make it an expensive affair. The classic low-carb keto foods, like meat, leafy vegetables, and high-fat fish can be expensive. However, for every one of the expensive ingredients, there are high-quality alternatives and substitutes that you can cook with that keep in mind the nutritional requirements of keto.

Keto on a diet simply needs a bit of ingenuity and planning to get it done. By the end of this chapter, you will know how to eat a high-quality ketogenic diet on a budget. With some of the money-saving tips already discussed and the insights you will get here, you should hack the keto diet on a budget.

There are so many tricks available to you, like buying supplies in bulk, looking for deals and discounts, and shopping at farm markets, which guarantee you savings and will easily support you if you are on a budget.

The benefits of keto diet on a budget:

- You will be able to stay on the diet despite low finances.
- There are still high-quality recipe alternatives and substitutes.
- Saves you money.
- You will still get the required calories and macros.
- You do not have to strain financially.
- No stress from lack of money to by the high-priced recipe items.

6.1 How to Succeed on a $50-a-Week Keto Meal Prep Plan

Here are some great ideas to help you to achieve a keto meal prep on $50 for a week of keto meals:

- **Plan in advance.**

Apart from keeping your meal plan simple, this is the most important point for cost-saving. Planning will save you money through the whole process—from purchase to restocking.

Planning prevents impulse and unnecessary purchases because you will have to shop as per a predetermined list.

- **Opt for cheaper ingredient alternatives or substitutes.**

Always go for cheaper recipe alternatives to the more expensive seasonal or classic recipe ingredients. There are high-priced and low-priced items for each food or ingredient category.

- *Cheese*

    This is a staple of the keto diet. Avoid specialty cheeses and buy a block of regular cheese and grate or shred it yourself.

- *Fish*

    Fish is a high-quality and healthy keto fat and protein source but is often expensive. Use canned fish in place of fresh fish if you are on a diet.

- *Poultry*

    If you have to buy chicken in parts, go for the cheaper cuts like thighs, legs, and wings. Alternatively, buy a whole chicken which is cheaper than buying parts.

- *Meat*

    Go for fatty meat cuts. They are cheaper than lean cuts, and buy from a butchery rather than a supermarket.

- *Vegetables*

Vegetables are integral to the success of the keto diet. Buy frozen vegetables instead of fresh low-carb vegetables, which are usually expensive at supermarkets. Frozen vegetables are cheap and do not go bad as fast as fresh vegetables.

- *Eggs*

    Stock a lot of eggs in your pantry. They are one of the cheaper protein sources and are versatile for keto recipes.

- **Shop in bulk.**

There is no better way of saving money or working within a budget that shopping for ingredients in bulk because it is cheaper. Stock up items on sale every time you come across them.

- **Be on the lookout for price discounts and offer.**

If you are on a budget, be on the lookout for price reductions and deals on quantities. This is a great way of getting more for less.

- **Avoid impulse buying.**

Simply put, do not purchase anything that you do not have on your shopping list; otherwise, you will mess up your budget.

- **Buy items online.**

Items are generally cheaper online. Take advantage of online stores to save money and get more items for at your weekly budget. You will be amazed at how much you save and get by buying things online than at the local supermarket.

- **Keep your meal prep simple.**

The simpler your keto meal plan is, the cheaper and easier it will be on your finances.

Tip: Do not buy a product or ingredient you have never used before in bulk because it may not be what you like or want. Buy a little to try and only buy in bulk if it is something for you.

Quick Start Action Step

Sticking to a keto diet on a $50-per-week meal plan is possible. You can even spend less depending on your preferences and meals choices. Use the insights in this chapter and take the simple options above to keep you healthy on keto when you are on a budget.

Chapter 7
Keto Meal Prep for Weight Loss

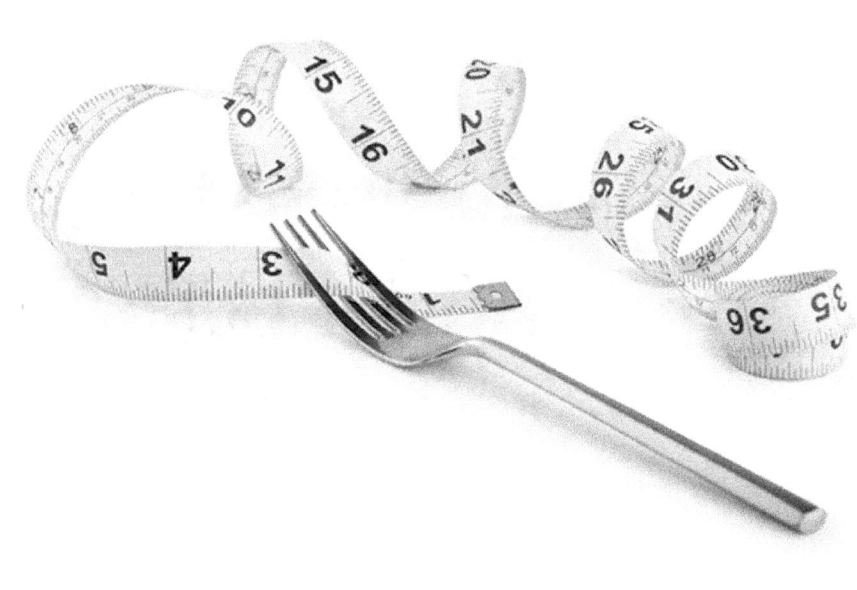

Chapter 7: Keto Meal Prep for Weight Loss

Just as you can do keto meal planning on a lean weekly budget, you can do the same for weight loss. A tight budget cannot prevent you from getting ingredients focused on weight loss.

As you are now aware, the ketogenic diet can be used for putting on weight, for maintaining the weight you are at, or for losing weight. For each of the three options, there are different and specific keto calories and macros that are effective and recommended for desired results.

Fat burning for weight loss is one of the main benefits of ketosis and is probably the reason why it is so popular. Keto makes people feel great and more satiated, which helps you to eat less of what you should not eat. It elevates mental and physical energy, which should not be impeded by low finances.

Achieving weight loss through keto on a lean budget is possible, and you should still be able to buy the weight-loss ingredients within your budget. Much of it is similar to what we have discussed in the previous chapter but directed at keto items for weight loss.

There are many keto weight-loss recipes and ingredients that can be cooked and bought respectively without spending so much money. Since dieting is about nutrition content in an ingredient of food, you will find nutrient-rich foods that are not necessarily in the high-price bracket. Make your pick from the list of affordable keto weight-loss ingredients further down.

7.1 Benefits of Keto Meal Pep for Weight Loss

The following are the foremost benefits of keto meal planning for weight loss:

- It elevates mental focus and concentration.
- It is highly effective at burning fat.
- It infuses your body and muscles with energy.
- It curtails constant hunger pangs.
- It helps in blood sugar balance and regulation.
- It improves skin health and fights acne.
- It controls cholesterol and triglyceride levels.
- It improves hormonal regulation in women, especially for severe PMS symptoms.

7.2 Affordable Weight-Loss Ingredients for Keto Meal Prep on a Budget

The following are great affordable keto weight-loss ingredients for one on a budget:

1. *Avocado*

Avocado is a ketogenic diet essential for healthy fat content, minerals, and vitamins. Not only is it good for its rich fat content but it also helps keto beginners to deal with symptoms of keto flu. It is high in fat and very low on carbs.

2. *Kimchi and sauerkraut*

Fermented foods carrying good bacteria, and prebiotic fibers are good for gut health. Studies have found that a healthy bacteria balance in your stomach can help to reduce fat mass.

3. *Eggs*

Eggs are the most versatile keto foods and one of the healthiest proteins for weight loss. Eggs will leave you feeling full and will keep you from packing extra calories.

4. *Garlic*

Garlic, as you know, has many long-exploited health benefits. A study found that garlic can help with weight loss.

5. *Leafy vegetables*

Collard greens, kale, spinach, and Swiss chard are great and affordable keto weight-loss foods. They are high in fiber, which slows digestion and iron nutrients which helps the body absorb the nutrients efficiently.

6. *Nuts*

Nuts are high in healthy fat and are not fattening as you may think. Look for recipes that incorporate them. Nuts improve metabolism and help with weight loss because of the high fiber content, which leaves you with a feeling of being full, thus keeping you from eating. Here are the best nuts:

- Almonds (carbs: 6 grams)
- Brazil nuts (carbs: 3 grams)
- Cashews (carbs: 9 grams)
- Macadamia nuts (carbs: 4 grams)
- Pecans (carbs: 4 grams)
- Pistachios (carbs: 8 grams)
- Walnuts (carbs: 4 grams)

7. *Protein powder*

Use protein powder to complement and supplement protein in your meals. Get protein benefits without extra calories—no extra fat or carbohydrates.

8. *Vinegar*

Use vinegar to replace high-calorie additions or condiments to your food.

9. *Pasture-raised chicken*

Eat free-range chicken and benefit from the fat-loss benefits of protein.

10. *Cruciferous vegetables*

Vegetables such as broccoli and cauliflower fall in this group and are keto staples because of their weight-loss benefits. They are a source of sulforaphane and fiber. Sulforaphane has been linked with stimulating energy-burning brown fat and improving gut health. It is also linked to fighting obesity.

11. *Olives and olive oil*

Olive oil helps with fat loss and promotes a leaner body. The healthy fats in olive oil and its anti-inflammatory properties are key to weight loss.

12. *Chilies*

Chilies have fat-burning properties, which are why obesity is low among people who consume a lot of chilies. Chilies contain capsaicin, which reduces appetite and boosts the burning of body fat.

13. *Coconut oil*

Coconut oil has healthy fats and promotes fat loss. A study of obese men found that supplementing their diet with two tablespoons (30 mL) of coconut oil daily helped them cut their waistlines by one inch.

These are some of the top keto ingredients that you can get easily when you are working with a tight grocery budget to help you with keto meal prep for weight loss.

Quick Start Action Step

Pick some of these keto ingredients to help you make the most out of your keto meal prep for weight loss.

Chapter 8
Keto Meal Prep—Mistakes to Avoid

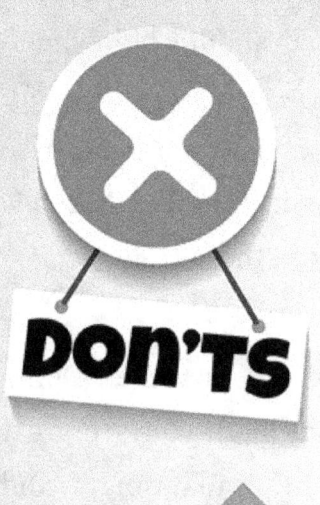
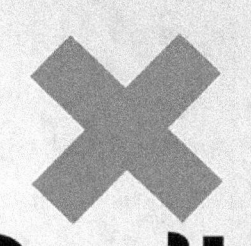
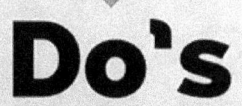

Chapter 8: Keto Meal Prep—Mistakes to Avoid

There are some common mistakes that people make on the keto diet that should be avoided because you will never succeed if you keep them up. In fact, it is possible to make some of these mistakes without knowing it. Keto meal prep is really effective if you stick to the script.

Keto does not have to drain your wallet. Doing things the correct way will help you see great returns on investment. Planning and preparation are key to making keto meal prepping very easy, and it ensures success.

8.1 Common Keto Mistakes

The following are some of the common keto meal prep mistakes you want to avoid:

1. Lack of Proper Planning

We already discussed the importance of planning for keto meal prepping. Lack of planning means that you open the doors for many things to go wrong. Failing to prepare means you should prepare to fail.

If you do not plan, you will eat the wrong things, waste time, and lose value for your money. An essential part of planning is doing extensive research into the ingredients and recipes you want to cook.

2. Eating Too Much Protein

You know the macro ratios required for successful ketosis. Eating too much protein is very easy and is a common mistake that must be suppressed. Too much protein consumption leads to elevated blood sugar because it is converted into glucose and defeating ketosis.

3. Low Mineral Intake

Ketosis increases acid production in the body, which lowers the body pH. Basic food minerals help balance out this state and create a normal pH.

4. Not Eating Enough Fat

Keto relies on fat for body energy; if you do not eat enough, you are putting a strain on the body, especially because you have cut on the other energy sources of the body.

5. Tracking on Carbohydrate Intake

Many people quickly forget that they should be tracking everything they eat and only track carb macros in the endeavor to reduce the carbs they consume. When you track only one macro, it is very easy to overeat another.

6. Eating Too Much Unhealthy Fat

As much as the keto diet is high-fat, consumption of too much of the wrong fats is wrong. Eating too much unsaturated fat should be avoided.

7. Not Drinking Enough Water

It is very easy not to drink enough water, and this is a common mistake by many people, especially newbies to the keto diet. Water is a must for keeping your body healthy while on the journey to ketosis and to maintain it. Dehydration while on ketosis can lead to kidney problems or failure. Put water at the top of your list.

8. Eating Only Animal Products

The efficacy of the keto diet can be misleading if you are not well informed. Include all food types, especially healthy vegetables. Plant foods are important sources of phytonutrients, vitamins, and fiber.

9. Eating Too Much Dairy Products

Consume dairy in moderation of on a keto diet. Dairy products are high in calories, which is counterproductive to what you want. You should burn more calories than you consume.

Forgetting physical exercise

Do not forget as much as the keto diet if efficient at burning fat. Exercise is important while on a ketosis diet to stimulate muscle building and calories and fat burning.

Bonus Chapter Money-Savings Tips When Shopping

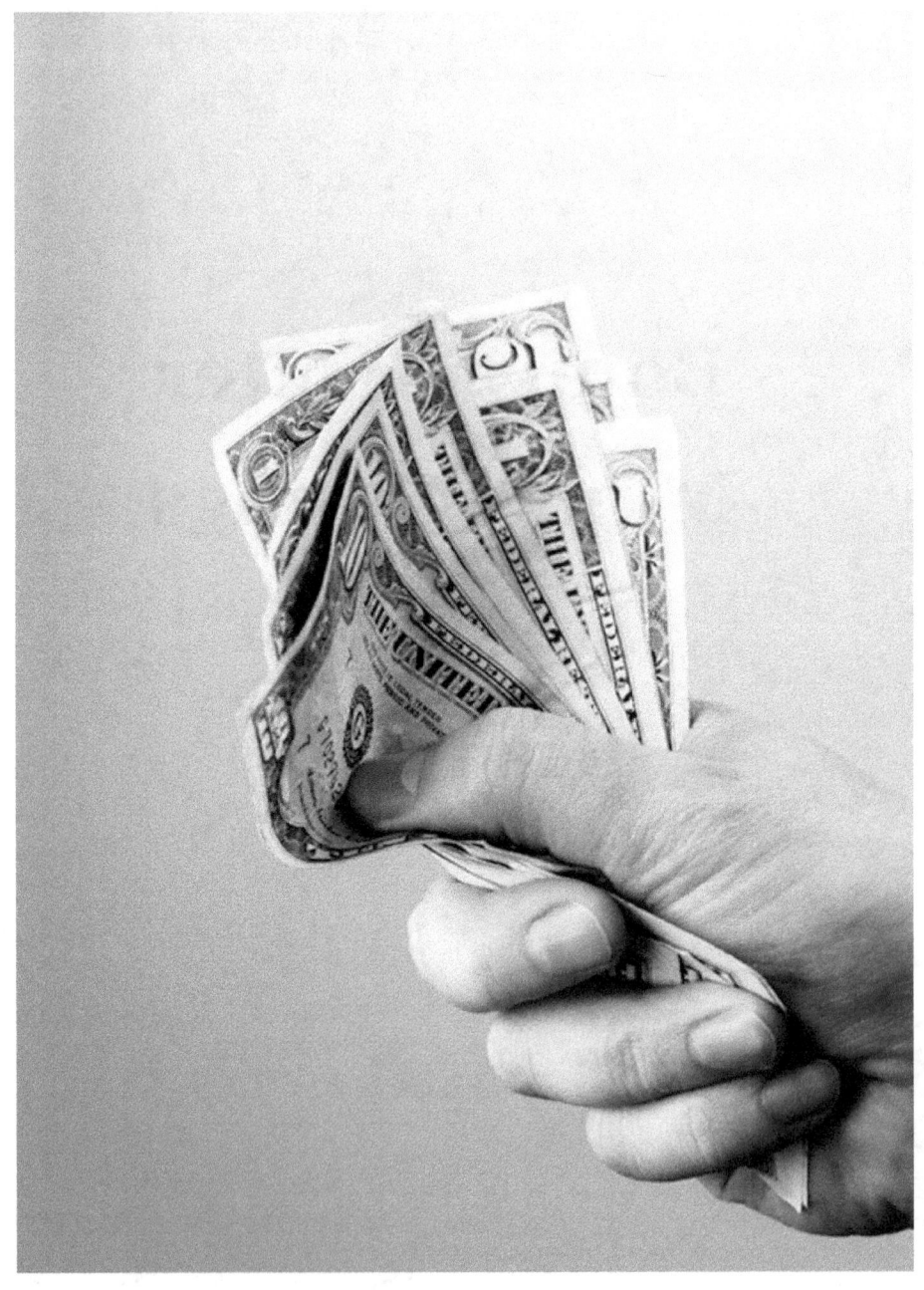

Bonus Chapter: Money-Savings Tips When Shopping

Here is a summary of keto meal planning money-saving tips when you go shopping:

- Much like shopping for everything else, making use of sales. Special discounts and coupons will save you a lot of cash.
- Buy items in bulk, enough for every week's meal prep; they will be cheaper. Also, refrigerate and freeze items just long enough to use.
- If you can, grow some of the vegetables you use on your own. It is much healthier and, of course, cheaper.
- Go for seasonal produce (fruits and vegetable) because they are cheaper and are more likely to be on sale.
- Shop at the farmers market for dairy, fruits, meats, and vegetables.
- Always go for fresh products. Avoid packaged produce because of the extra expense you will incur.

- Keep your meal plan simple. The fewer the ingredients you require for your meals, the less money you will need to buy them.
- Go for frozen vegetables when fresh options are not available.
- Always buy a whole chicken and cut it yourself. Buying cuts is expensive.
- Make most purchases when there are price deals, such as discounts and clearance sales.
- Shopping online is cheaper.

Preview Of 'Keto Diet for Beginners: Your Ultimate & Essential Step-by-Step Ketogenic Lifestyle Guide to Losing Weight Fast and Eating Better for Long-Term Weight Loss, Healthy Living and Feeling Good' by Amy Maria Adams

Chapter 1: Getting Started with the Keto Diet for Beginners

1.1 Definition of the Keto Diet

The ketogenic diet, also called the keto diet for short, is simply a diet that is high in fat and low in carbohydrates. It is also sometimes called low-carb, high-fat diet, or simply low-fat diet. The diet aims at reducing the intake of carbohydrates and replacing them with fat; this has many health advantages. By reducing the consumption of carbohydrates, the body is put in a metabolic state known as ketosis which is an increase in the number of ketone bodies in the blood.

When on a ketogenic diet, the body initiates a natural phenomenon in order to help us survive whenever food intake is low; this leads to efficiency in the way the body burns fat for energy. Also, fat is turned into ketones in the liver, which supplies energy for the brain; this is because the body is naturally adaptive to whatever is put into it. When there's an overload of fats and a reduction of carbohydrate intake, the body then begins to rely on ketones as its primary source of energy.

1.2 Benefits of keto diets

The ketogenic diet differs from other diets in the sense that many of those diets offer weight loss as their main advantage. The ketogenic diet comes with a large number of benefits because of the way it alters the chemical composition of the body. The keto diet leads to an increase in the production of ketones, as well as a dependence on ketones for the daily maintenance of the body. The body is more efficient when it depends on ketones as fuel. Amongst the many advantages of the ketogenic diet, a few will be discussed below:

• **Weight loss** – because of its low carbohydrate content, the ketogenic diet brings about a breaking down of body fat into ketones and allows the body to depend mainly on ketones rather than glucose. In other words, the fat stored up in the body will be used as a source of energy. When an individual is on a keto diet, insulin, which is the fat-storing hormone level, drops massively, turning the body into a fat-consuming machine since fat storage is prevented. Scientifically, on long-term analysis, a regularly practiced ketogenic diet has proven to show better results as compared to low-fat and high-carb diets; cholesterol is produced from the conversion of excess glucose in the diet. Ketogenic diets generally have an improved feeling of satiety, hence leading to an overall reduction in food intake. This allows for reduced calorie intake without necessarily causing ravenous hunger.

- **Reversion of nephropathy** – nephropathy is one of the complications associated with individuals who have uncontrolled diabetes. Studies have shown that keto diets aid the reversing of diabetic nephropathy by increasing the level of 3-beta-hydroxybutyric acid in the blood, which leads to the subsequent reduction in the metabolism of glucose in some tissues within the body, for example, the kidneys. In a study performed by Poplawski et al., during one week of administering the ketogenic diets to rats, the glucose level in the blood normalized. Within two months, the albumin/creatinine ratio was also standardized, and diabetic nephropathy was completely reversed. This is associated with the expression of genes induced by oxidation and various forms of stress being normalized. In a human, the ketogenic diet causes a decrease in the level of creatinine as compared to the consumption of low-calorie foods, which show an increase in the level of creatinine. Ketones can serve as an alternative source of energy.

• **Boost brain health** – the brain, unlike the muscles, cannot utilize fat as a source of energy; therefore, the brain is heavily dependent on glucose. The brain, however, can utilize ketones. The liver uses fatty acid to produce ketones in situations where glucose and insulin levels are low. Ketones are usually produced in little amounts when one hasn't eaten for long hours, for example, after a full night's sleep. However, the liver's production of ketones increases during periods of fasting, starvation, or when the level of carb intake is below 50 g per day. When the consumption of carbs is minimized, ketones can cater for up to 70 percent of the brain's needs. Although most of the brain can utilize ketones, some parts depend solely on glucose for their functionality. When one is on a low-carb diet, some of this glucose can be provided for by the small intake of carbs. The body, however, synthesizes most of the glucose requirements in a process known as gluconeogenesis. In this metabolic process, the liver produces glucose for the brain to utilize; it uses amino acids as its raw material. The liver can also produce glucose from glycerol; this is the backbone that connects fatty acids in triglyceride molecules—the body's form of storing fat. Staying on a ketogenic diet has been proven to be effective against Parkinson's disease as well. It is most likely that certain features associated with remaining on a ketogenic diet, such as an increase in brain sharpness, mental clarity, and less frequent migraines are related to the controlled level of sugar in the blood serum and change of energy source for the brain, which helps improve memory.

- **Increase in the levels of HDL cholesterol** – whenever people hear about an increase in the level of cholesterol, there is usually a panic, and this is because many are not well informed that there are two types of cholesterol (the HDL and the LDL). The HDL is the one that is more needed because it carries cholesterol from the body to the liver (the liver is where it can be reused or excreted.) Conversely, the LDL transports cholesterol from the liver to all parts of the body.
- **Reduction of epileptic seizures** – seizures are a complication associated with epilepsy. It usually manifests as continuous jerking movements and fainting; it occurs mostly in children. Epilepsy is tough to treat. There are several types of seizures. Although many effective anti-seizure medications exist, these drugs are usually ineffective in at least 30 percent of epilepsy patients. This type of epilepsy is known as "unresponsive to

medication." The ketogenic diet, developed by Dr. Russell Wilder in 1921, supplies the body with about 90 percent of calories from fat and is effective in treating drug-resistant epilepsy in children, as it has been said to imitate the important effects that starvation has on seizures. The particular mechanism, however, remains unknown, but it is believed to help in increasing the stability of neurons and regulation of mitochondrial enzymes.

- **Beneficial for individuals with Alzheimer's disease** – ketogenic diets provide benefits to people with Alzheimer's disease. Alzheimer's is a gradually advancing disease in which the brain develops tangles that result in loss of memory. Many researchers believe that it should be classified as "type 3" diabetes because the brain cells develop insulin resistance and lack the ability to utilize glucose properly, causing inflammation. Health experts claim that Alzheimer's disease has certain common features with epilepsy, for example, overexcitement of the brain cells that leads to seizures. It has been suggested that ketogenic diets may be an effective method of fueling brain cells affected by Alzheimer's disease. One hypothesis is that ketone bodies protect the cells of the brain by limiting the level of reactive oxygen species which are by-products of metabolism that may cause inflammation. Another hypothesis states that the lethal proteins that accumulate in the brains of individuals with Alzheimer's disease can be reduced by a diet that contains a high amount of fat.

• **Battling cancer** – cancerous cells express a metabolism that is different from the metabolism of healthy cells. They are usually characterized by rapid increase in glucose utilization. This is due to the many insulin receptors in them, causing them to thrive in an environment that has high levels of both insulin and blood sugar, usually caused by mutations and mitochondrial dysfunction. Cancerous cells, unlike healthy cells, cannot effectively utilize ketone bodies as an energy source. Also, ketone bodies restrain the proliferation of tumor cells, and they can provide energy for healthy cells without feeding the tumor cells. Ketogenic diets, however, can only be helpful against some types of cancer.

• **Boosts energy levels and improves sleep** – after staying on a ketogenic diet for about four to five days, most individuals experience an increase in energy levels and a general lack of interest in carbohydrate diets; this is as a result of a readily available energy source and the insulin level being stabilized in body and brain tissues. When placed on a low-carb diet, the body can only store so much glycogen, and as a result, constant refueling is necessary to maintain energy levels. However, your body already has as alternative fat storage to utilize; this means that ketosis is a source of fuel to the body that can never be exhausted and you'll find that you have energy throughout the day. The mechanism of sleep improvement remains a mystery. However, studies have shown that staying on a ketogenic diet helps improve sleep by reducing REM and increasing slow-wave sleep patterns. This is most likely related to the biochemical shifts associated with the brain now depending on ketone bodies as an alternate energy source and other body tissues breaking down fat. However, during the first few weeks of staying on a ketogenic diet (the adjustment period), you may experience particular difficulties in staying asleep and insomnia. This will wane with time as your body becomes accustomed to ketosis and to consuming stored-up fat. And then you'll find that you feel more relaxed, can sleep deeply for more hours, and feel rested when you wake.

• **Aids kidney functions** – kidney stones and gout are mostly caused by an increase in uric acid, phosphate, and calcium levels. This is as a result of obesity, dehydration, consumption of sugar (especially fructose), and alcohol consumption. Uric acid levels can be temporarily increased by ketogenic diets, especially when a person is dehydrated, though its level decreases over time. Uric acid levels increase within the same time frame as ketone bodies, but after a period of four to six weeks, uric acid levels begin to decrease despite ketone levels staying up. Hence, the individual might have a low uric acid level despite being in a state of nutritional ketosis.

• **Helping women's health** – polycystic ovary syndrome (PCOS) can be effectively treated with low-carbohydrate diets which help to stop specific symptoms such as obesity, infrequent menstrual periods, and acne. Keto diets also help in keeping the level of sugar in the blood serum deficient and stabilized. They also help to maintain the level of other hormones, and especially in women, this has a lot of benefits in a wide variety of metabolic pathways associated with insulin.

• **Helps battle type 2 diabetes** – individuals that suffer from type 2 diabetes exhibit excessive insulin production. Because keto diets are low-carb and hence remove sugar from the food, they assist in the reduction of the HbA1c count. That can, therefore, help reverse type 2 diabetes. Ketogenic diets also help in reversing nephrology, provide cardiac benefits, assist with weight loss, and improve lipid profiles.

• **Helps boost gastrointestinal health and liver health** – it is common knowledge that grain-based foods, nightshade vegetables (such as tomatoes, potatoes, etc.), and sugar-filled foods increase the chances of heartburn and acid reflux. It is, therefore, of little surprise that maintaining a low-carb diet helps improve these symptoms, confronting the problems of autoimmune responses and inflammation. With regards to this, changes in diet alter the total human gut microbiome (you are what you eat). A variation in the microbiome substantially reduces most gastrointestinal problems as a result of staying on the ketogenic diet. Studies have shown that carbs in the diet are highly associated with gallstones as they are the main ingredients that cause them. As a countereffect, eating an appropriate amount of fat when carb intake is down assists in the clearing out of the gallbladder and improves functionality, thus reducing the chances of gallstones forming. Fat accumulating in the liver is related to prediabetes and type 2 diabetes; in very extreme cases, fatty liver disease can be very lethal to the liver. This condition is usually tested using a blood test to measure the level of liver enzymes.

- **Decreases inflammation** – ketogenic diets are highly anti-inflammatory and help in improving a lot of health problems. The anti-inflammatory properties of ketogenic diets, or a reduction in caloric intake, may be linked to retardation of the hormone responsible for inflammation. In other words, the main ingredients responsible for most inflammatory diseases are repressed by ketone bodies made from a ketogenic diet. Thus, its effect on acne, psoriasis, eczema, arthritis, and other inflammation-associated diseases is reasonably significant enough to attract more research attention. It is, therefore, very possible to improve a whole host of conditions through nutritional ketosis.
- **Helps in appetite control** – when staying on a low-carb diet, you'll find that you don't feel hungry as often as before; you don't develop random cravings that make you go on an excessive snacking spree and cause you to eat bad things. Many individuals that stay on a ketogenic diet find it easier to perform intermittent fasting, where you're feeding not as

consistently as before, and you only get to eat at certain set periods of the day. Controlling the sugar level in the blood can help with curbing such cravings and uncontrollable appetites.

This book will help every newbie understand the keto diet; there are recipes within the book to try out which will improve your health and well-being.

1.3

One of the ways you can find out how much you know, do not know or need to know about the keto diet as a beginner and is to take online tests. That's a good way of checking your knowledge base (if it's sound enough) and there are many websites where you can take such tests. You can take tests at "Completely Keto" at http://completelyketo.com or "Bhu Foods" at http://bhufoods.com

Your Quick Start Action Step:

Create some time before the end of the day to take the test at any of the websites listed above and take the tests.

None of the tests should take more than 15 to 20 minutes.

Chapter 2: The Ketogenic Diet – Common Questions Answered

2.1 Is the ketogenic diet safe?

It is normal that whenever a new diet hits the scene, there's always information that talks about its negative impacts on your health. However, what is the case with the keto diet? The keto diet has undergone scientific tests and analysis and has been recommended by great medical institutions globally. It has been proven to be safe; however, this depends on the activity level and condition of the individual. But on a general scale, it is entirely safe. It is helpful for achieving a healthy lifestyle and not just a miracle cure.

2.2 Does the ketogenic diet work?

The ketogenic diet has been in use for a very long time; it became more pronounced in the 1920s and since then has been used repeatedly on different individuals. The keto diet started as a cure for epileptic children, with many of them being completely cured. The ketogenic diet has been proven to work for many conditions starting from weight loss to heart disease. Its impact on weight loss has been debated as a short-term impact; some patients apparently regain weight after about a year or two. But this is highly debatable.

2.3 Does the ketogenic diet work for the long-term?

It is highly debatable whether the use of ketogenic diets for weight loss works for the long-term; however, it is not medically or scientifically proven otherwise. Using weight loss for other diseases works, for example, for people with diabetes, and the cure is long-term. The same thing applies to high-blood pressure if they are able to follow through with the diet successfully.

2.4 Does the ketogenic diet affect weight loss?

The answer is yes. The ketogenic diet is gaining popularity again not precisely because of its benefits for other diseases but because of its use for weight loss. The ketogenic diet is beneficial for weight loss because of the dramatic reduction in the intake of carbohydrates, forcing the body to burn fat as its source of energy rather than glucose from carbohydrates. It also reduces appetite, which also contributes to weight loss. By affecting appetite, it reduces individuals' cravings for sugar.

2.5 How does a ketogenic diet affect cholesterol?

It is a common misconception that since ketogenic diets are high in fat content, they lead to an increase in cholesterol levels in the body. However, this is not true. Much scientific research has shown that low-carb diets help in optimizing the cholesterol level in the body.

Many are unaware that there is good cholesterol and bad cholesterol. HDL cholesterol is the one known as "the good cholesterol." It collects all cholesterol that is not in use within the body and takes it to the liver, where it is either recycled or destroyed. The ketogenic diet causes a reduction in LDL, "the bad cholesterol," which is responsible for some cardiovascular diseases in adults.

2.6 What is the "keto flu" and how do you minimize it?

Starting a keto diet can be very strange. You have a lot to look forward to including a lot of weight loss and a lot of anticipated internal changes that your body is bound to undergo. However, keto flu is something else that might also come along when starting a keto diet. Your body may experience keto flu during the initial stages of being on a keto diet. Usually, the body gets a little weak before it finally starts getting stronger. The extent to which your body suffers usually depends largely on your previous diet as it determines the shock your system will undergo from your new diet pattern; the effect of that shock is what you will begin to experience.

Once you start a keto diet, some symptoms are sure markers of having the keto flu. They include:

• Headaches

• A cough

• Fatigue

• Irritability

• Nausea

These symptoms are usually indications that your body needs to adjust to the changes in your diet pattern and adapt to what you're putting it through. Having these symptoms is not enjoyable, and it sucks; they can leave you discouraged and make you wonder whether it is worth the pain and discomfort. However, these symptoms will eventually fade away as your body approaches ketosis. These symptoms are just your body reacting to carb deprivation, but over time, these symptoms will go just as quickly as they came.

A ketogenic diet contains a very low-carb content, and therefore your body tries to adapt to the low intake of carbs since you have been consuming a large amount of carbs your whole life up to this point. Staying away from carbs will tend to come as a shock to your body, but very soon your body will recover and continues on the path to good health. When suffering from the keto flu, you may start to consider eating more carbs to make the pain and discomfort go away, but do not listen to this temptation; endure for a couple of days, and everything will go back to normal.

How to minimize the flu?

Once on a keto diet, one of the numerous changes your body will undergo is a loss of body fluids and electrolytes in the form of sodium, potassium, and magnesium. Electrolytes are vital to the proper functioning of your body as they play a significant role in determining the amount of water in your body and how effectively your muscles perform their task. Carbs usually help with water retention within the body, ensuring there is no excessive loss of electrolytes. When staying on a keto diet, you will begin to lose a lot of body fluids, and since most electrolytes are dissolved in these fluids as a solvent, it is natural that you will lose some of them. Also, since your body is going to be consuming a lot of stored-up body fat, and your body cells will begin to replace these fats with water, it is essential to stay hydrated. It is also necessary to add a lot of salt to your daily meal by eating foods that have a high sodium content. If your electrolyte consumption is high, then you'll be just fine.

How long will it take for my body to adjust?

When on a regular diet, your body is, necessarily, sugar dependent but when on a keto diet, your body becomes fat dependent. This kind of change usually has a drastic effect on the body, but time is all your body requires. The adjustment period differs with individuals.

However, on average, it takes more than a week to finally reach the ketosis stage; for some, it occurs faster than that. It all depends on how your body reacts to the effect of such changes; this is the time your body begins to shed some fat. It is essential to note that even when your body has reached the ketosis stage, that doesn't mean it will stay in it when you begin to eat carbs again. Some individuals can get away with it; others can't. It is just safer to adhere strictly to your diet.

2.7 How many carbs can I eat on the keto diet?

The amount of carbs every individual needs is dependent on a couple of things. Generally, eating less carbs has more impact. It will speed weight loss and reduce appetite and hunger. Someone with type 2 diabetes should eat fewer carbohydrates; it will improve insulin resistance. The truth is that many people find a diet that is very low in carbs somewhat too challenging and restrictive.

2.8 How much protein should I eat on the

keto diet?

When on a keto diet, it is essential to eat a lot of protein. However, if you eat too much of it, this will lower your ketone levels; if you eat too little, it leads to you losing excess muscle. So you should be at the midpoint in that sense. For someone that is sedentary, that is, you do a whole lot of sitting during the day, you should eat around 0.6 grams and 0.8 grams of protein for every pound of lean body mass. If you are someone who has an active day, you should eat between 0.8 grams and one gram of protein for every pound of lean body mass. If you want to gain some muscle, you should eat about one gram and 1.2 grams of protein for every pound of lean body mass. You don't need more protein than that.

2.9 What ketogenic diet is best?

In selecting the best diet, there are some things to consider. If you're someone who rarely engages in highly intense exercise and wants to lose weight, you should stick to the standard keto diet. If you add more carbohydrates, you will only be slowing down your progress and prolong how long it takes to reach ketosis, unlike those who don't add carbs. For people who engage in intense exercise regularly, then the cyclical keto diet and the targeted keto diet might be right for you. If you're someone who has only started intense workouts regularly within the last year, you should try out the targeted keto diet and see if you notice a decrease in performance while you're on the standard keto diet. When it comes to figuring out the best type of keto diet for you, it is important that you experiment. There are no individuals that are the same; you must find out what works for you best. It is important also to note that if you're not doing intense exercise regularly, then you should stay on the standard keto diet. Usually, most people do not need anything more than the standard keto diet.

To learn more about this book and how it can help you achieve a healthier lifestyle, look for the title "Keto Diet for Beginners: Your

Ultimate & Essential Step-by-Step Ketogenic Lifestyle Guide to Losing Weight Fast and Eating Better for Long-Term Weight Loss, Healthy Living and Feeling Good" by Amy Maria Adams on the online store.

Measurement Conversions

Liquid Volumes		
mL	US	fl. oz.
5	1 tsp.	
15	1 tbsp.	1/2
30	1/8 c.	1
60	1/4 c.	2
78	1/3 c.	
118	1/2 c.	4
158	2/3 c.	
177	3/4 c.	6
237	1 c.	8
355	1 1/2 c.	12
474	2 c.	16
710	3 c.	24

946	4 c.	32
When exact measures aren't necessary, you can round 1 c = 250 mL.		

Dry Weights	
Grams	**Ounce to Pounds**
28	1
57	2
85	3
113	4 oz. = 1/4 lb.
151	1/3 lbs.
227	8 oz. = 1/2 lb.
302	2/3 lb.
340	12 oz. = 3/4 lb.
454	1 lb.
907	2 lbs.

Oven Temperatures	
Celsius	**Fahrenheit**
140°	285°

150°	300°
160°	320°
170°	338°
180°	356°
200°	392°
220°	425°
225°	437°

Conclusion

Thank you again for owning this book!

I hope this book was able to help you to help you understand how to do keto meal planning successfully. We defined what keto meal prepping and planning is and delved into the benefits of adapting meal planning for the keto diet.

Further, we looked at the steps required of proper meal planning and went through what you need to do from start to finish. By now, I am confident that you know the essentials of keto meal prepping for your pantry and kitchen. You know how to shop and the right containers to store your food for the week.

We did not stop there, we looked at the importance of macros for keto meal planning and got insights on how to calculate macros and why we should.

This book has dedicated two chapters to keto

recipes. Chapter 4 carries simple and easy go-to keto recipes for keto meal plan beginners while the next chapter is a reservoir of great keto meals that will keep you excited about meal planning for months.

More importantly, chapters 6 and 7 look at how to shop for keto ingredients on a budget, which is important because a lean budget should not hinder us from achieving and maintaining ketosis.

The next step is for you to take the insights and tips from this book and ingratiate them into your keto meal prep plan. The benefits are numerous, and the joy you will get from the information and the recipes in this book is invaluable.

Thank you and good luck!

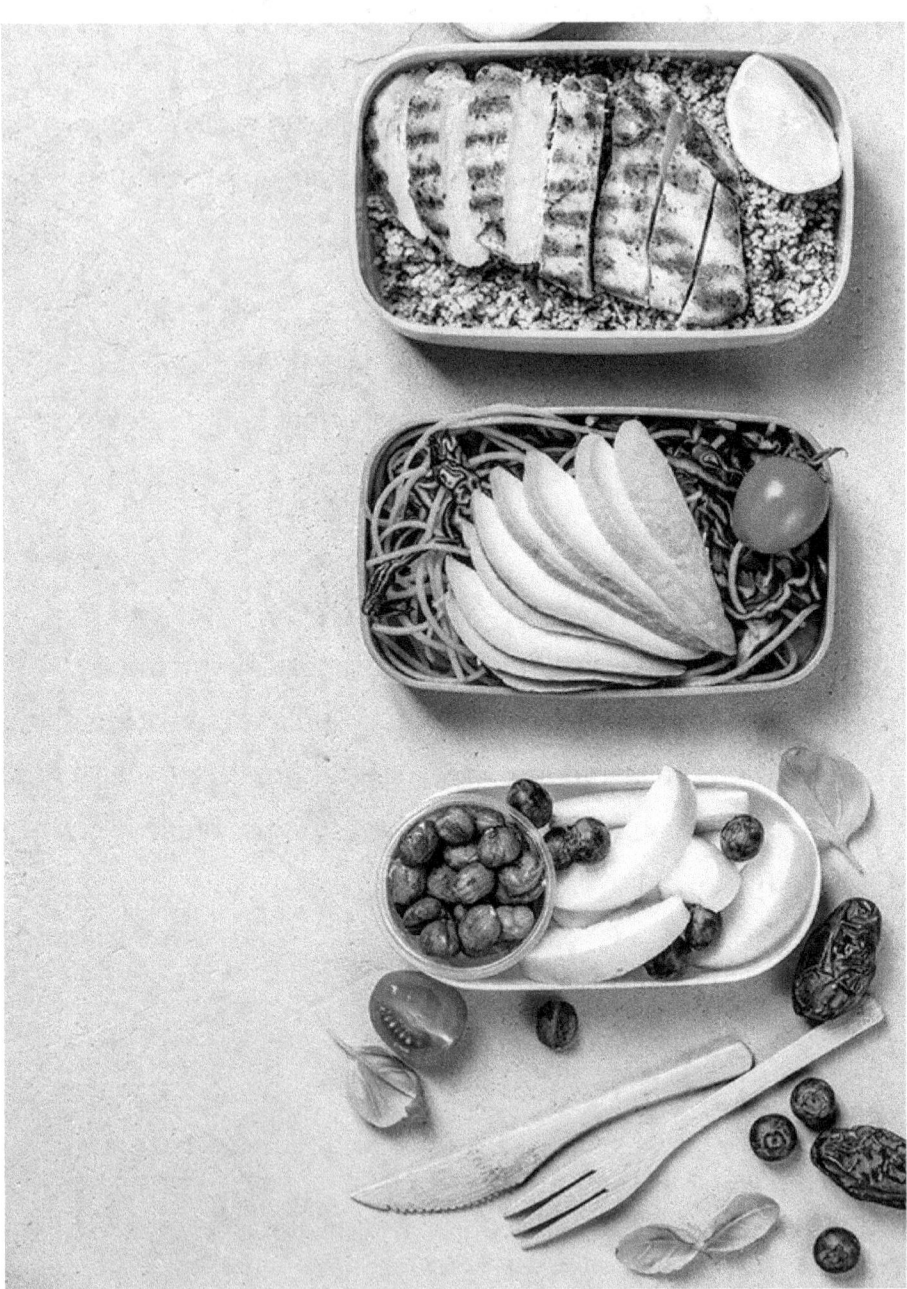

www.ingramcontent.com/pod-product-compliance
Lightning Source LLC
Chambersburg PA
CBHW071229070526
44583CB00017B/2105